Rebuilding the Body After Chemo, Radiation and Surgery

Wellness = nutrition + supplements + detoxing + exercise.

DIANA WRIGHT

Doctor of Naturopathy
B.S.N., M.B.A., A.A.D.P.-B.C.

ISBN 978-1-7372784-1-2

For more information, address: diana@dianawrightnd.com

First paperback edition May 2021.

Book design by Taisa O. Palmeira

For more books and award-winning film, *The Unbelievable Plight of Mrs. Wright*, check out Diana's website www.dianawrightnd.com.

LEGAL NOTICE:

The information provided in this book is intended to educate the reader about certain medical conditions and certain possible solutions. It is not a substitute for examination, diagnosis, and medical care provided by a licensed and qualified health professional. If you believe you or your child or someone you know suffer from the conditions described herein, please see your health care provider. Do not attempt to treat yourself, your child, or anyone else without proper medical supervision.

DISCLAIMER OF LIABILITY:

The materials in this book are provided to you "as is" without warranty of any kind, either expressed or implied, including, but not limited to, the implied warranties of merchantability, fitness for a particular purpose, or non-infringement.

My belief is that the body is stressed with an accumulation of environmental and internal factors that prevents the body from healing. As these factors are removed from the body, the body can heal itself as God intended.

In no event shall Diana Wright, her staff, heirs, or assigns nor Private Membership Association, nor Divine Health or their associates or employees be liable for any damages or incidental damages or damages for loss of profits, revenue, use or data, whether brought in contract or tort, arising out of, or connected with this book or the use, reliance upon, or performance of any material contained in or accessed from this book or our website.

Your reading of this book implies that you agree to the release of liability noted above.

INTRODUCTION

The mortality rate among cancer patients is very high. Naturopathic therapy cannot be a substitute to the standard chemotherapy and radiotherapy but can be used in combination with cancer therapy to decrease the side effects of the drugs.

The body can heal itself when all the underlying issues are corrected. God has miraculously made the body this way. With each layer of illness that has healed, we can then move on to a lower layer to heal. It is like peeling away the layers of an onion.

Synergy is when a person combines traditional medical treatment with alternative treatment for a Total Treatment for cancer and advanced diseases. We know that one thing did not cause the illness, so you must do more than one thing to be well. It is critical to recognize that this is not an all-or-nothing approach. The same is true in reverse. Too many patients and healthcare practitioners separate natural from allopathic (traditional medical treatment) therapies, and do not give enough emphasis on the practicality of using both together.

Cancer organizations statistics on the mortality rate of cancer proves that traditional therapies aren't successful. The difference is alternative therapies aren't dangerous. Even if they fail, they aren't going to add to the problem or kill you. Unlike chemotherapy and radiation, your body will not be a wasteland after a failed naturopathic treatment.

There are many thousands of testimonials from people on the Internet claiming that natural therapies for cancer cured them. These people are not trying to get rich as they are not trying to sell a product. These are legitimate medical "miracles".

I have learned from my own Stage 4 (late end stage) cancer journey that a cancer patient should use multiple effective treatments when treating cancer. I recommend if they use frequency generating devices, they should also include nutritional protocols. Through the synergy of multiple strategies, individuals can create an inhospitable environment for cancer in their bodies.

Remember advanced Cancer will kill you for sure.

Cancer remains the second cause of death in America after myocardial infarction.

After a body has had chemotherapy, radiation or surgery and considered healed it is time to rebuild.

TABLE OF CONTENTS

CHAPTER 1

"He will wipe every tear from their eyes. There will be no more death or mourning or crying or pain, for the old order of things has passed away."
- Revelations 21:4

Controlling your blood glucose and insulin levels through diet, exercise, emotional stress relief and mediation or prayer are the most critical components of any recovery program.

I was given only eight months to live by MD Anderson, the cancer center at the University of Texas, but was told that I probably wouldn't live even that long. I had ovarian cancer of the uterus, both ovaries, the omentum, rectum, colon, vena cava, aorta, and to top it off, I had three brain tumors, as well. MD Anderson said that I was terminal. But other than God, who really knows? Here I sit writing this, 9 years later.

I transformed my body, turning it into an inhospitable environment for cancer to grow. The first thing I did was to change my body chemistry to an Alkaline pH to control cancer while I researched how to make the lifestyle changes necessary to return to good health.

I used both allopathic and naturopathic means to reverse and to prevent metastasis and to control metabolic disturbances. After years of treatment, I underwent another surgery on October 23, 2015. Three doctors thought that I had another brain tumor, while one thought that what was present on the MRI was old damage. There was no brain tumor.

The surgery left me unable to walk or talk. Just like the 46 other misdiagnoses, the surgery was an abysmal mistake. All this took an incredible amount of perseverance. After all that I was forced to suffer through, what I learned was that Allopathic Medicine had betrayed me. There was not a chemical panacea for every malady. With that, I decided to become a Naturopath in 2018 and be the custodian of my own health. And that's exactly what I did!

I own a machine that produces alkaline water, and an ozonator, that produces ozone (additional oxygen). Cancer and advanced disease cannot grow in an oxygen-rich environment. Every day, the water I drink is first accessed through the alkaline water machine with an alkalinity of 9.5; I then run this water through the ozonator. According to Jensen, "Ozone contributes to greater oxidation in the human body and functions as an antiseptic and tonic for the body."[1] To stay in perfect health, the range of both the Urine and the Saliva must be a 6.4 pH.[2] I use pH test strips to verify the amount of alkalinity.

MY STORY

Unlike most people, I know exactly the day my cancer started. January 2, 2011, my entire office decided to go on a diet together, as we had worked hard. I rewarded them all by taking them on a cruise. My large staff (www.therightsolutions.com) is a rather unusual, as there is a strong sense of fellowship and love for each other, and because of this, many of us choose to do things for group support, such as dieting together. We had all decided to start on the HCG diet and lose weight for our cruise. We all wanted to look our best in swimsuits. According to Dried Blood Cell Analysis, "Every day, the body is fighting a war. It is fighting a battle for survival against our environments and our own lifestyles."[3]

HCG, THE PREGNANCY HORMONE

HCG is a human gonadotropin hormone. It is the pregnancy hormone that allows a baby to grow in our bodies without consuming it. HCG is the hormone that differentiates the sex organs of the baby, without which, the baby would not grow into a normal fetus, as the body would gradually devour it through the immune process. HCG also stimulates the hypothalamus to secrete fat stores into the bloodstream; this is how the diet works. Unfortunately, cancer utilizes the HCG hormone to hide, according to Ralph W. Moss, PhD:

"Cancer and pregnancy share a number of characteristics, one of which is an altered immune system. In pregnancy, the embryo, which is biologically distinct from the mother, must find a way to avoid being attacked as a foreign or non-self-mother's immune system. HCG appears to have a role in making the embryo invisible to the mother's immune system, and may play a similar role in cancer too, disguising the immunologically foreign characteristics of the tumor in such a way as to prevent the immune system from recognizing and challenging the abnormal cells."[4]

But I didn't know all this the day that I started on my HCG diet. I also didn't know that I had a genetic condition (BRCA1), which predisposed me to cancer.

Within a few days of beginning the HCG, I started hemorrhaging, and would continue to do so for 40 days until the diet was over. I made an appointment with my oncology gynecologist to find out why I was bleeding and he ordered a pelvic ultrasound, which he pronounced clear. The radiologist did not agree, but I didn't ask for my test results, trusting my doctor. I didn't know of my condition until I was diagnosed with stage IV ovarian cancer—a terminal diagnosis. Trusting my doctor to do the right thing and actually READ the report was an error that nearly proved fatal!

THE METABOLIC DISTURBANCE

As I progressively got sicker and sicker, I looked for more and more doctors, had more and more tests, and was consistently misdiagnosed. Not one of the doctors discovered that I had ovarian cancer. I would have to conduct research, make inquiries and undergo testing which seemed interminable, until my diagnosis was finally conclusive. Making one wrong diet decision had changed my life forever. Over the next year and a half, I saw 6 different doctors and had 45 visits with failed diagnoses.

To cope with my failing health and reduced energy levels, I increased my coffee intake, which only made my body more acidic. I used alcohol to come down at night, further increasing my body's acidity. I already called stress "my drug of abuse," which also made my body very acidic. The combined acidic toxic slew consisted of HCG, stress, alcohol, caffeine and coffee, processed flour and sugar, table salt, black tea, fried foods, unclean foods, empty foods, processed oils, anger, an improper relationship with God, and worry. This combined to create the optimal environment for cancer growth. As I put single cation substances into my body, it created a low-energy, highly acid environment, and my illness grew.[5]

I had bone degradation, weight gain, fungus of my head, thinning of the skin, bladder and kidney problems, periodontal gum disease, intestinal polyps visible on a Colonoscope (I was diagnosed with both rectal and colon tumors), depression, anxiety, and nervousness.[6]

I exercised and ate two salads of raw food daily. The biochemical induction was not enough to combat a body that was predisposed to cancer through the genes I possess. I had both the MTHFR genes, (A1298C double mutation, and C677T double mutation) and BRCA1 (2798, del 4). I have a COMP gene for increased anger as a byproduct of my higher intelligence, entrepreneurial ability, and ability to perceive stress as less than others might. Green Tea turns this "on" and "off" through epigenetics. I need this ability to run my large business. I threw the Green Tea away.

THE ILLNESS

I was so terribly ill over the year and a half leading up to the diagnosis that I was constantly visiting allopathic doctors. I even had my breast implants removed because I was concerned that they were contributing to my illness. During this time, I did not miss work or any family activities.

In April of 2012, my stomach inflated, making me appear six months pregnant. My husband and I noticed it, and worried about my weight—which had not increased—but we didn't think about cancer.

In May 2012, I went to lunch with my assistant—a beautiful, super-efficient lady named Maureen who had worked with me for years. I started having chest pains during lunch but thought it would clear up. It didn't. After lunch, I visited the nearest doctor's office. Dr. Jonathan Parker immediately gave me nitroglycerin, which provided immediate cardiac relief. I asked for another one and Dr Parker got nervous. No one ever wants a second dose of nitroglycerin. He immediately sent me to the closest hospital, Washington Regional, where I was admitted to the cardiac ward. Because I was in perfect shape, I was monitored and tested and declared to be cardiac healthy. The hospitalist said that I had Esophageal Spasms. Esophageal Spasms! Ridiculous! I knew that that diagnosis was not accurate but still did not know what was wrong with me. Because my personality is to leave no stone unturned, I made an appointment for an EDG and a colonoscopy even though I was not due for a colonoscopy for 3 years. Dr. Rogers saw a large ovarian tumor through the colon wall. He took biopsies of the colon wall, which were negative, of course. I thank God, in his error, the doctor did not perforate the colon wall to rupture the tumor. After 2 weeks, I was a nervous wreck and still had no definite diagnosis.

The "benign" colon wall biopsies were a gross error, but the doctor did not think he needed to order a Cat Scan. This situation was ridiculous. I had top-of-the-line insurance, money to buy my own Cat Scan machine if I wanted to own one but was hassled when I requested that one be performed. I returned to Dr. Parker to request a Cat Scan, and the results were definitive for ovarian cancer.

THE DIAGNOSIS

June 28, 2012 was a date that rocked my life and the life of everyone close to me. When you receive a terminal diagnosis, it not only affects the life of the person that is diagnosed, but of everyone in your family, close friends, neighbors, co-workers, church members and many people you didn't even realize cared. My diagnosis was like that. People cared. Some people cared a lot.

I would learn that not everyone acts as you would expect when they deal with your illness. I sat up all night sipping cake vodka and crying over the prospect of facing the end of my life. I had one fantastic pity party. I had worked so hard to come from a terribly abusive childhood, to overcome a lack of education by obtaining a GED, to work so hard to get a bachelor's degree in nursing while working full time as a single mother. I worked day and night to be happily married, and to take care of family members who were ill and dying (while I was still in my twenties and thirties), all the while raising children of my own. I worked hard to get my master's degree in business and to win every business award under the sun. To compensate for the mental and physical abuse I endured as a child, I excelled in my work. My goal was never again to be poor or mistreated. I had spent the last seventeen years building my dream business, starting alone in the beginning until I was eventually running a multimillion-dollar business with many dear, hard-working employees. My company had come though the recession with fantastic success where so many other companies had failed. Under my leadership, TRS had thrived. Was this how all the hard work was going to end? Was I going to be cheated out of enjoying the fruits of my labor? Was this it? These feelings were incomprehensible and heart-rending.

My fourth daughter, Ali, drove home immediately to go through the testing with me. She insisted that I go and pick up the results of my Cat Scan. The gift of Ali has always been interesting. I say the "gift of" Ali, because she was always truly a gift to me. Ali was my brother's child. He and his wife could not get their lives together, so I took her as my own.

Ali is a very low-key person who rarely expresses her thoughts but has always been there when I needed her the most with sound advice.

As the all-day testing was scheduled, it was a rush to work in a trip to medical records in between the tests. Ali was insistent. We had to have a copy of the Cat Scan! I was complacent. I didn't understand it then, but I had started on a path that would last at least a month when I lost interest in food, life and everything around me. Cancer patients need to have an advocate that takes charge and manages the medical plan because you just cannot process it. I am a super-competent, organized, high-energy person that gets more done in one day than most people do in a month. But at that time, I just could not function.

At Ali's urging, at 1:25 we were at Medical Records and they gave me copy of the film on a CD but refused to give me the written report that the doctors had in hand the day before. I was immediately suspicious. I know that the report is available on the computer and is a quick printout. When I questioned the two clerks from Medical Records, they flatly refused to answer. I called my sweet Dr. Parker across the street from my office and sent my son-in-law, Jay, to run over and get the reports. It was Friday afternoon and the doctor closed at 1:30, but Dr. Parker stayed open long enough for Jay to get a copy of the report.

We did not finish the testing until 4:00 in the afternoon. We stopped by the office to get the report and as I pulled out onto the highway, Ali said, "Mom, you've got to read this report. This is not right." As I was driving, she tried to interpret the results. I could not understand the horror she was saying. I had to wait until we got home (where Julia, my third daughter, was waiting for me), to read the report myself.

As I walked into my kitchen at 4:20, my mind would not process the Cat Scan report. I could not believe what I read. The Oncologist, for whatever reason, had lied to me and my family about the severity of my disease. I had a 7.5 cm left ovary tumor, a rectal tumor, a colon tumor, tumors throughout the peritoneal cavity, uterus and smaller right ovary and the omentum. He had failed to mention any of this except the left ovary and the colon.

Let this be a lesson to everyone. Always get the test results! They belong to you and you paid for them. If ,for any reason, they do not want to give them to you, you must insist! I almost let a man who lied to me operate on me. If I had, I would be dead today.

CANCER AND THE PLAN FOR SURVIVAL

My life as I had known it was over. I was a planner and thinker. I always had a plan for everything. But not cancer. It was just too big. Too much.

When I found out I had cancer it felt as though a ton of bricks had fallen on me. I was stunned, bereft, incredulous, and overwhelmed. I could not function. I could not think. I could not stop feeling that my life had been upended. I soon found out that shock, depression, and fear would become part of my daily life for the next six months until I developed a plan for survival and the eradication of cancer, but not myself. The acidity of my body contributed to the escalating emotions in this crisis.

There had to be an answer somewhere. But what? I received a call from a stranger named Lydia, a cancer researcher. Lydia said many things to me, but the one that I remember most was "you only have one opportunity to get surgery right. Go to a major medical center and get the right diagnosis, get the right surgery, and the right treatment. You cannot redo a wrong surgery."

Within minutes of Lydia's call, my nephew Kevin came to be there for me. Kevin is a 30-year-old licensed minister. He is sensitive, kind—an exact copy of my personality—except without my temper and caustic side. A perfect being. He sat with me that Saturday morning and we discussed the phone conversation that I just received from Lydia. The choice was "Go for treatment" or "Stay in Northwest Arkansas." This was the issue that I could not wrap my mind about. He prayed for me. I felt better immediately with the prayer.

WE ALL **THINK** WE HAVE A VOICE (BUT WE REALLY DON'T)

Soon my family and friends started showing up. All things in my life seem to come in clusters, and this catastrophe was no different. This weekend was the weekend my second daughter, Melanie, and her husband Clint, had sold their home and were moving to Stillwater, Oklahoma, where he was to start his new job as a college professor. They were to sign the paperwork to sell the house on Friday morning, spend that afternoon and evening cleaning the house, spend the night in a hotel Friday night in Bartlesville, Oklahoma, then drive to our home Saturday morning. Melanie and Clint have two boys, Sawyer, 3, and Beau 1, and Melanie was pregnant with their third son who was due in January. Melanie's birthday is July 1.

I realized that we needed to have a birthday party of some sort, as the family was going to be together that evening. I am a gourmet cook, and throwing together a party in 30 minutes had always been my specialty, but that day, I could not function. We planned a party anyway. But not everyone was invited—this was to be family only. We had to talk about the business and what to do.

As the afternoon progressed and the family and close friends assembled, it was readily clear that the divided camps had even more clearly split. After the conversation with Lydia, I decided to go to MD Anderson immediately. It was surprising to me was that my husband and I were not on the same page. As the debate continued, it became clear to me that I had decided about my care, but for some reason all the people closest to me felt they were entitled in the name of love to make decisions for me. I had never lost control of my life before, so it was time for me to get it back. I would take responsibility for my own medical care.
I told them I was going to MD Anderson for testing immediately and it was

definitive. I have never been a wishy-washy woman. I was strong. I guess too strong. My husband said I needed to go down there by myself and be a big girl. The conflict continued until my best friend Christy said I could not go alone, and I had to choose someone to go with me.

JULIA

Julia, my third daughter, is super calm and speaks in a very calm soothing voice. Julia and I had worked together for years. We had perfect harmony when dealing with other people to get the results we needed. Together, we thought outside the box, I was outspoken, and verbalized our injustices while she calmly and reasonably talked the offending party into correcting the issue. Together we thought of all possibilities. She was the only person who could help me face this decision. She and I work together in perfect sync. Julia was also six months pregnant with my second granddaughter.

That night, as the family gathered for the very sad group birthday party dinner, many decisions were made concerning the business. My son-in-law, Taylor, would assume the role of CEO; my son-in-law, Jay, would assume the credentials manager role; and my niece, Amy, would assume my husband's CFO role. This would free my husband to be my caregiver. Just the idea that I might need a caregiver was so depressing and sad. I realized that my self-sufficiency may be pushed to the limits over the next few months if I survived at all. But the blessings that I had in my daughters, my sons-in-law, and my sweet niece made my life worth living.

I spent all day July 3, 2012, with Julia, being tested and seeing my assigned MD Anderson Gynecology Oncology Doctor. Many of the tests were a repeat of tests that I had done in Arkansas. MD Anderson doesn't recognize testing from other hospitals on initial diagnoses. The test results confirmed the ovarian cancer and resolved the issue of the chest pain. I had cancerous lymph nodes on both my vena cava and my aorta.

EMOTIONAL UPHEAVAL

Overnight, my personality and demeanor completely changed. I went from being a very strong, emotionally secure, articulate, fun-loving and happy CEO to withdrawn, emotionally volatile, and sad. My husband and I had always been of one mind. We were closer than close, but on this issue, we were not at the same place. My husband distanced himself as he tried to come to terms with this situation. I consider myself a realist—David would say I'm negative-focused—but how can you optimistically look at Stage IV cancer? When I get upset, David usually responds by downplaying the situation. He always thinks that this is going to make me feel better, but it really makes me feel panicked; I don't trust his judgment and I think that things are worse than they really are. Even though we've been married 40 years, we still operate in this manner. It makes both of us crazy as he downplays, and I escalate. You'd think we'd learn to handle things a little more constructively.

I always think of relationships as an emotional bank account. When you have a negative interaction, it takes five positive interactions just to be back at a zero balance. Because David and I had years and years of love, honesty, and friendship, we had an emotional bank account with millions of emotional points stored up. My philosophy on my husband was always to treat him better than anybody else in the whole world. I truly tried to live up to my wedding vows of love, honor, and respect for my husband. But we just couldn't agree on how to handle this tragedy. I began to feel replaceable by the distance that cancer was causing in our relationship.

One morning, as we were preparing to go to work together, he made a comment on the financial impact that the cancer might have. This is a perfectly innocent comment by my husband, as he has always paid the bills, been responsible for investments, balanced the checkbook, and while we both earned money, I earned more than my share. My temper flared, and I fired at him, "I don't know why you're worried about it, you're going to get everything—the house, the money, everything, and a new wife. Win, Win, Win for you and I'm going to be dead." My husband's much too smart a man to say a word, he just looked at me sadly. But this was a pivotal point for our relationship; he had to get on board with me and help me look for a cure. I had been so strong in my life, founding and building a company from scratch, taking care of all the family, and everything else I had done to be successful. But I just couldn't do this by myself. I needed my husband to continue being the partner he had always been.

STARTING LIFE AS A CANCER PATIENT

When I got ready to leave on Sunday, July 16, 2012, I was able to report out to Taylor, my son-in-law, in four hours, on a company I had taken 16 years to build. Truly life was becoming more and more distressing as I felt increasingly replaceable.

As I prayed about my diagnosis, I got a clear message from God that I was to do whatever anybody asked of me, take any medicine (natural or chemical) that I was told to take, and do everything that anyone brought to me to cure my cancer. On my last day at work, there was a line out my door and down the hall, of people who cared about me, bringing me everything they could think of to save my life. The accounting manager's cousin, Marcia, showed up in my office with a Kangen water machine that filters city water and turns it alkaline. It is critical for cancer patients to drink alkaline water, as healthy cells regenerate at a pH of 7.88 which is an alkaline environment; it produces a lactic acid environment. Most cancer patients' bodies are acidic as a result. Marcia also gave me the book by Robert Wright, Killing Cancer, Not People. A local pastor and his wife brought me Barley Life and Proancynol 2000 for colds, both AIM products. These are wonderful body balancers. Barley Life is also alkaline producing. One of my employees brought me Quartz Crystals to put in my pillow. My Recruiting Manager brought me a juicer which creates juice full of enzymes that are alkaline producing. All vegetables are alkaline producing.

My last day as CEO was a full one. The next day, I would become just another cancer patient at MD Anderson. Once you become a cancer patient at MD Anderson, you forfeit your identity. You become a number, very much like a holocaust prisoner. Your number is your identity. I was number 069716.

HOUSTON

David and I packed the car for our several-month stay in Houston. As we drove, I read Robert Wright's book, Killing Cancer, Not People. I had never been a cancer expert, never worked on oncology, and really had not given a lot of thought to it. I knew my father's family had more than its share of cancer deaths. My aunt Carolyn died at the age of 38 to "stomach cancer." That was a lie told to me as a child, so I wouldn't have any sexual thoughts. My aunt died of ovarian cancer. If I had ever been told that a first-degree relative had had ovarian cancer it would have raised my level of awareness as a registered nurse, and the level of awareness of all healthcare professionals that I had visited.

My father died of esophageal cancer. My favorite aunt, his sister, Alma, died of breast cancer. Alma first had breast cancer at age 30. Back in the 1950s, she was treated with radiation and surgery. She lived cancer free but very sad, until the age of 56 when her husband died, and her immune system bottomed out and the cancer came raging back, Stage IV. Both my father and his siblings had the same genetic cancer I had. One of my brothers died with cancer.

Robert Wright's book gives you perspectives that are not common in the allopathic medical community. I am allopathically trained with a registered nursing degree. I was horrified when I realized that I was going into a chemotherapy program where my five-year survival statistics were only 2%.[7] I realized right then that chemotherapy alone would not save me.

I knew that chemotherapy alone would not cure my cancer. I knew that I was going to have to come up with a plan—a comprehensive alternative plan—to support my immune system that the chemotherapy was designed to destroy. Only a complex approach to stop every possible way that cancer attacks would even give me a hope of survival. 75% of women with ovarian cancer die within the first year. One thing alone would not cure me. Of that I was certain.

TESTING AT MD ANDERSON

Our first week in Houston, Texas was a rough week. We would get blown out of the water with a horrible diagnosis of bone cancer, to be told later that it was not bone cancer but an old back injury. I was sent for a mammogram, rushed to a sonogram, had an emergency ultrasound of the breasts only to be told there was nothing wrong.

I had an 18-inch needle biopsy of the left ovary with no anesthesia. To get to the left ovary, the doctor entered my right side, *for his convenience*—he couldn't be bothered to walk around—and drove the large bore needle all the way across my abdomen to the left ovary. It was unconscionable! I had to submit to this procedure with no pain medication. The pain was unbearable—the most horrible, excruciating pain I have ever experienced. The biopsy shot my CA 125 cancer number through the roof! My CA 125 went from 350 to 758 overnight! The cancer was growing out of control, caused by the rupture of the tumor by the needle biopsy. **Beware of biopsies. The only reason they are needed by the doctor is to provide documentation to the insurance company.** This week was truly a roller coaster of emotion for both of us.

EDUCATING MYSELF

David and I went to Barnes & Noble and bought every book they had on cancer. We purchased over 20 books that day. I had to get educated to save my life. As the CEO of a large company, I was used to strategic planning. According to Dr. Barry Richardson, Dean of the College of Business at Centenary College, in Shreveport, Louisiana where I received my master's of business degree, "You can be an expert on anything in one week." I knew this was true as I presented paper after paper in MBA school on industries, of which I knew nothing about a week earlier. I got to work. I read the books, I wrote plans, I Googled everything I didn't know, and I self-educated on what was available in the United States. Soon it became evident that the only thing available was chemotherapy, radiation, and surgery. Effectively, the allopathic medical community had moved so far away from proven effective methods of treatment that the current treatment appeared ludicrous. There had to be a chemical pill for everything. You were considered lucky to be accepted into a trial.

As I got more educated, I got more depressed. There were so few options available in America. Almost none. There were no good options available for me. There were no solutions. Nobody had a cure for stage IV cancer—in the United States, anyway. The FDA has kicked it all out.

THE HORRIBLE DOCTOR

The second week we were in Houston began the realization that my doctor at MD Anderson was incompetent. She would walk into the room, rush around, drop a horrible bomb such as "You have stage IV cancer," and run out the door before I had a chance to ask any questions, ignoring me. This behavior became the norm. My doctor's behavior continued to deteriorate over the following eight weeks while she conveniently disappeared on "vacation". But when she was there, she consistently refused to answer any questions and dashed out of the room immediately. Her favorite quote that she used every single time she saw me was, "I can get you in remission if YOU decide to respond to chemotherapy." Blame the patient. The oldest trick in the book for a poor physician with no people skills. I had known all my medical career that a doctor with a poor bedside manner gets sued more frequently than a physician that has lesser skills but a great bedside manner. In hindsight, I am so glad I was assigned a poor physician, or I would have stayed at MD Anderson and probably would have died there.

PROTOCOL VS. SENSITIVITY TESTING

MD Anderson is supposed to be the leading cancer hospital in the United States. However, instead of treating cancer individually according to a sensitivity test to see exactly what kills the cancer, which is a routine protocol for bacterial infections, they use a "standard written protocol."

No wonder so many people have such poor outcomes with chemotherapy. The patients are receiving chemotherapy that is not toxic to their cancer, but is instead, toxic to their immune systems. Doesn't it make sense that you should use the chemotherapy specifically targeted to kill that specific cancer? It does to me. But at that point, I wasn't aware of chemotherapy's sensitivity testing. For all my nursing career, all hospital patients with infections were sensitivity tested to see what antibiotic would work best on their infections. But in America, with chemotherapy, we do not run sensitivity testing. It is simply not done.

Suzanne Summers' doctor, James Forsythe, runs this test routinely and has it processed in Greece. It is all detailed in her book, *Knockout!*

THE GIFTS OF CANCER

Dr. Bill Tim, my Naturopath, sent me a liquid multivitamin, as well as calcium, magnesium, and zinc supplements. According to Bernard Jensen, Ph. D, "Alkalinity of blood and lymph are increased, and every cell is saturated by these (vitamins). Heart action is supported, arterial pressure stabilized, and circulation is promoted by potassium."[8] Melanie, my second daughter, found a licensed physician in Houston who heals doing energy work through laying on hands and prayer. She worked on me three times and I do believe that my healing is directly related to her work through God's will. She sent me to a Chiropractic Doctor who got me started on the right supplements to balance my body. He drew my blood which was extremely thick as the alkaline water was causing my cell debris to increase and be forced into my blood. This was due to alkalizing my body. According to Analyzing pH, "increased salts cause severe heart stress with thick blood."[9] According to Dried Blood Cell Analysis, "Blood is a liquid substance that has three general functions: transportation, regulation, and protection. By circulating minerals such as calcium, chloride, and potassium, the blood is able to regulate pH."[10] Water intake was increased. I tested several times per day using Litmus Paper, and if the pH was acid, I drank baking soda mixed in water to increase my alkaline levels and get rid of cancer.

The supplements, energy work, diet changes, positive mental changes, decreased stress, and clean lifestyle changes worked together to help protect me from the side effects of the chemotherapy. I didn't suffer from all the terrible side effects that the patients around me were suffering from. However, MD Anderson gave the same misinformed axiom: "Take no vitamins that interfere with the chemotherapy." The staff have no idea which chemotherapy will kill the cancer because they chose not to do the sensitivity testing available in Europe, but they are sure the vitamins will interfere. I am sure that the vitamins I took did NOT interfere with the chemotherapy process, but instead, healed and supported my immune system during the chemotherapy process.

DIETETIC CONSULT

The MD Anderson dietician told me to go make milkshakes and make sure I matched all sugar with fat, like brownies, so I didn't lose any weight. I had been very diet conscious my whole life as a Registered Nurse. I knew better than to fill up on brownies and sugar. **Everyone knows that cancer is a metabolic disease and sugar is cancer's favorite food. That is how**

the PET Scan shows up cancer as it sucks up the radiated sugar, and lights up cancer like a Christmas Tree. Unnatural (manmade) sugars decrease immune system function. I wasn't about to help cancer kill me by eating sugar.

STARTING CHEMOTHERAPY

Chemotherapy started on July 27, 2012. I woke up that morning with a terrible feeling of dread in my stomach before I ever even got up. I knew I would survive chemotherapy that day, but at what terrible, terrible cost? I had to go to the lab first so that my doctor would have an accurate blood count to order the chemotherapy. Another protocol. This one, however, made sense, as chemotherapy cannot be given when your blood counts are too low—a side effect of chemotherapy. Today, however, was my first day, so my blood counts were unimpaired.

David and I waited two hours after the lab for our appointment with the doctor to see if the chemotherapy would be ordered that day. The doctor behaved as usual, answering no questions, being very short and abrupt, and leaving us totally bewildered. From there, we went to the chemotherapy ward where we waited for over five hours after our scheduled appointment time before we were called back for chemotherapy to begin. The area that we waited in was attached to a lovely rooftop garden, full of beautiful flowers. I wandered through the flowers for over four hours. David sat inside and waited for my name to be called. He was so kind. I was totally overwhelmed with the imminent end of my life. At this point, we had been at MD Anderson since seven that morning and it was 3:30 in the afternoon. They still hadn't started chemotherapy. All this waiting caused extreme anxiety, which increased acid, which in turn exacerbated by already overwhelming emotional state. I was so distraught, it was a blessing when they finally gave me so many drugs, I passed out.

I found a shriveled flower that appeared to be dying and put it in a plastic zip lock bag. I had put it in my purse. I knew that one component of fighting cancer was to visualize your body fighting cancer and winning. As they started the IV, dripping all the pre-medications into my body, then finally starting the toxic Carboplatin and Taxol, I looked at my dried-up flower and I visualized my ovarian cancer shriveling up and dying. I visualized all the blood vessels feeding the cancer shriveling up. I visualized myself getting stronger.

The next week, when I pulled out my flower from my purse, there was a hideous bug trapped in the bag. I had never seen a bug like that in my life. It was so terrifying to look at, and I knew it was a sign the cancer was receding. I pinched it dead.

Blessedly, I passed out quickly with the pre-medications each time I received chemotherapy. So, the time went very fast for me, but very slow for David. But he never left my side and he never complained about the time that he spent with me. It was after 9 PM before we finished chemotherapy and went home that first night. Our first chemotherapy session lasted over 14 hours. We both left emotionally devastated, and physically exhausted, and feeling as though this was one of the worst experiences of our entire lives.

THE DAY AFTER

The morning after my first round of chemotherapy, I felt terrible. But the most amazing thing happened. Starting in April, my belly had started to swell, although my weight did not go up. We discussed if the changes in my body were just part of menopause. That morning, instead of a six-month pregnant belly, my belly was almost flat. It was shocking and proof to both of us that something must've happened to shrink the tumor on the day after with the first dose of chemotherapy.

I had artificial nails on my fingers. They had told me at MD Anderson these had to come off. I soaked my nails that morning in acetone to remove them. The acetone contributed to the heavy metal poisoning of the carboplatin and Taxol. This was the absolute worst chemotherapy session that I have ever experienced. My stomach churned for days. The Zofran did absolutely nothing to control the nausea. My horrible doctor refused to write me a prescription for Emend, but she did write me a prescription for 1000, 4 mg Dilaudid. I also got a prescription for 600, 2 mg Xanax. When I looked these up, I found that both caused the immune system to be depressed. There is no way I was taking anything to depress my already low-functioning immune system. The chemotherapy was doing a good enough job of destroying my immune system without any additional help from me.

That afternoon, David's niece called and invited us to go to dinner that evening as her daughter was in a swimming competition close to where we were staying. Because I wanted gifts for the children, I decided to go grocery shopping before we went to dinner. David dropped me off and went to get gas while I ran into the grocery to pick up a gift for the children and a few other things. I had no idea the impact the chemotherapy had on me until I could not find my way to the front of the store to check out. I wandered around feeling sicker and sicker while becoming increasingly panicked. I had never had a feeling like that before. I was always in control. Here I was, lost in a grocery store! The impact of the poisoning of the chemotherapy was much greater than I had ever imagined.

CHEMOTHERAPY THE MD ANDERSON WAY

Chemotherapy was a weekly occurrence at MD Anderson. Needless to say, it was an abysmal experience. It was in a different place each time it was scheduled—never the same building twice. There was no continuity of care. You never saw the same nursing staff member but once, and I only saw foreign nurses. I was surrounded by people who were obviously dying, and in varying states of agony and misery. Chemotherapy side effects were poorly managed. The worst night I had, I was placed in a section with very few patients, so they decided to close the floor. I had so many drugs coursing through my veins, I was barely conscious. At long last, my foreign nurse, with a nearly undecipherable accent, entered the room and asked me to stand. I could not. His inability to communicate was alarming to me. How can one practice medicine in America without the capacity to speak the English language? This RN insisted that I walk to a building across campus about half a mile away. I flatly refused. I couldn't even stand up, but that made no difference to him. Very frustrated, he finally got me a wheelchair, but I was required to push my own IV pumps with six bags of fluid. Absolutely ludicrous.

THE ART OF WAITING IN IMAGING

Waiting at MD Anderson is an absolute art form. My doctor decided that I needed a CAT scan. I was to show up in the CAT scan department at 11:00 AM. We sat in a completely packed radiology waiting room on hard, plastic chairs. At 4 o'clock, people started to be called back and were asked to put on a gown. I am a small, slender woman, so the hospital gown wrapped nicely around my naked body. Other patients didn't have the same experience as way too much flesh was on display in the waiting room. As they sat with their naked rear ends on their hard, plastic chairs, I wondered at the total incompetence of the radiology department who acted as if they had never done this before. At 6 o'clock, they called each of us back—and there were hundreds of us—to put on a pair of scrub pants. We were then sent back to wait in the waiting room. At 9:00 PM—remember, I had an 11:00 AM appointment—I was called back, and instead of the cat scan, I got a MRI. Only after questioning the error, did I receive a cat scan. I was charged for both.

We didn't leave radiology until after 11 o'clock at night. We were totally exhausted, as our day had started with lab at 7 AM, a full 16 hours earlier!

HAIR – OR THE LACK OF HAIR

Chemotherapy continued. My days were filled with researching everything I could find on cancer. David's days were filled with working remotely for the company. We walked two to four miles every morning, and entertained ourselves in Houston with movies and museums. My research led me to believe that I needed to be on a very strict organic Modified Fasting Diet of fish, vegetables, and fruits. I eliminated everything else. My goal was to live in a healing, alkaline state. I tested my saliva and urine multiple times per day to make sure I was in a healing alkaline zone of 7.88 pH. The weight was falling off me. I started my trek to Houston, weighing 141 pounds. I was now losing a pound a day.

Weight has always been a sensitive issue for me. I watched my beautiful, lovely 38-year-old aunt who had cancer slowly starve to death until she weighed a mere 40 pounds. At the time she died, her beautiful face had been transformed into a skull with a thin layer of skin stretched over it. There was no resemblance of my beautiful aunt any longer, but more of a terrifying zombie. I can still see that face clearly today. I was 10 years old.

As the weight continued to fall off, my incompetent doctor just kept telling me, "Don't worry, it's all tumor weight." When I asked if that was a good sign, she said the same thing as always: "we won't know anything until we see how **you** decide to respond to chemotherapy." Always, all my fault! The medical doctor saw herself unable to cure cancer.

On August 1, 2012, my third daughter, Julia, and her husband, Taylor, came to Houston to accompany me to chemotherapy. As I was scheduled for chemotherapy late the next day, Julia and I decided to use the morning to go get my beautiful long hair cut off. David and I had bought 2 wigs earlier in the week. I had been hoping that my hair was at least 10 inches long, so they could donate it to Locks of Love—it was 12 ½ inches.

My hair was cut, leaving long bangs in front, with the rest of the hair was shaved off the back of my head. After only one week of chemotherapy, my hair was already falling out. I was told it would take 10 to 14 days, but this was not my case. My hair fell out in less than a week.

I had always been the woman who said that I was not my hair. I did not think that my hair defined me. I could not have been more wrong or more devastated when it fell out. God gave me the exact hair I was supposed to have because my life was so difficult, running my own business, raising the children, and being a wife. If I had any other hair, I would've never been able to make it to work on time. My hair was perfect for me. It was neither too thick nor too thin, it was straight but curled beautifully, and wearing it long, it was easy to pull up into a French twist which always looked classy for business. My hair was easy—being bald was not. It is not socially acceptable. People stared. Being bald is not comfortable. Wigs are scratchy, winter is cold, the summer sun burns you, and the wig makes you sweat. You really don't have a lot of options to look normal without a wig. I've heard lots of people say how cute scarfs look. I'm a woman who wore a scarf every single day of her life to work, around my neck. When I put a scarf on my bald head, I just thought I looked more sickly.

I think that's the biggest problem with being bald. You just look sick. When you look sick, you start feeling sick. When you start feeling sick, you start feeling depressed. When you start feeling depressed, you have anxiety over feeling ugly. When you look in the mirror and see the bald head, all you feel is depressed, anxious, ugly and sick. All this negativity combines to create more acid.[11] It's a vicious cycle, and there's no way out until the chemotherapy is over and the hair starts growing in again. There's no way to look normal even with a wig when your eyelashes and eyebrows are gone. The only upside to this is that the rest of your body is completely hairless also, and it rivals the most expensive Brazilian wax. I thought I might embrace my baldness. Boy, was I wrong.

My sweet husband would hold me at night and kiss my bald head and I would just cringe. Talk about a passion killer!

THE FIRST PATH TO HEALTH

David and I were emotionally falling apart at the seams. We were so low emotionally that grief radiated from us. One look from the energy physician, and she took us straight back to her office to talk to us. She absolutely radiates light. When you stand in her presence, you feel the presence of God. She is truly an angel. After two hours, she sent David to the waiting room, had me lie down on a patient exam table, anointed me with oil, and began energy work.

During this session, as I lay back, I immediately went into a semiconscious state while she prayed for me and went to work balancing my energy. I had never had any energy work done before. During this session, I saw my emotions bloom up as a yellow flower and explode in a hail of purple sparks. She saw exactly what I saw, and this bonded us. I was the only patient she had ever had this experience with. I still don't know what experience I had. But I would do it again in a second, because it relieved so much of my anxiety, grief, and near hysteria. She provided me with the impetus to regain control over my life, and started me on my path toward naturopathic healing.

THE POWER PORT

So, while my emotional self was coming back together, my bone marrow decided to fall apart. I had had one round of dose-dense chemotherapy, and my platelets, red blood cells, and white blood cells all took a beating. Dose-dense chemotherapy is when they take one chemotherapy round normally given every 21 days and give the Carboplatin in a full dose, with one third of the Taxol in week one, then give one third of the Taxol in week two and week three. This is better tolerated and easier on the patient. When I went for lab, I was unable to have chemotherapy on the day that I was scheduled. This turned out to be a blessing for me because this was the day that I was scheduled to have my subclavian port inserted into my chest without anesthesia.

At MD Anderson there is only one Doctor that surgically inserts power ports in every patient. Dr. Joe Brown had put in over 8,000 ports at the time that he saw me on August 16, 2012. Dr. Brown is very tall and thin. When he saw me lying in the bed, he remarked on what a tiny woman I was and that he would fit in the smallest power port available. When I had an anesthesia consultation for my port, I was told that 10% of all the women over 40 who have surgery at MD Anderson have brain damage from the anesthesia. I have no brain cells to spare. I was facing major surgery in October to remove the uterus, fallopian tubes, ovaries, omentum, appendix, with possibly a bowel resection, and rectal resection, I could not afford brain damage in August. I told Dr. Brown I would not be using anesthesia and I would lie still for the port insertion. I guess he saw I was serious because he did not question me.

As I was wheeled into the operating room with the sheets up to my chin and the lights blasting in my face, I was terrified. Dr. Brown slid into the operating room dressed in his operating gown, hat, and gloved hands in the air exactly like Tom Cruise slid into the room in the movie Risky Business. A big-screen TV lit up with karaoke songs. He burst into song. I could not believe that my doctor was dancing and singing "You're My Teddy Bear" to relax and entertain me. When the surgery started, he started singing songs appropriate to the situation designed to calm me down such as, "We're Supposed to Be Together".

I received a slight topical anesthesia and lay perfectly still while my port was installed in my right shoulder and the catheter ran down the subclabian vein down into my heart. It was sutured into my jugular vein. While I was distracted during surgery, I was in intense pain (It lasted for three weeks). I held my arm so still for three weeks that I created a calcification in my shoulder from the pain of the surgical site. In hindsight, I would have done it the same way because I still can't afford to have any additional brain damage.

I'll never forget the kindness and care Dr. Joe Brown gave me. I have had no problems with my port, and it has functioned perfectly. I really am glad the chemotherapy was canceled that day as I was so sick from the installation of the port, I really don't think I could have tolerated chemotherapy in addition to port surgery. The only three good things that came out of my time at MD Anderson was an accurate diagnosis, my incompetent doctor following allopathic protocol giving me carboplatin and Taxol as first-line chemotherapy, and the most excellent Dr. Joe Brown putting in my port.

THE REALIZATION

After four blessed days off chemotherapy, we started up again. By this time, I had read all 20 of the first set of books that we had bought on cancer and bought another 20 books. I was becoming more and more distraught over the dismal statistics with the poor outcomes of ovarian cancer patients. I found out that within five years, 98.1% of stage IV cancer patients who use chemotherapy alone, are dead. While I'm a risk taker, nobody in her right mind would take that kind of risk. Who would gamble living with less than a 2% chance? I started calling the oncology doctors that were writing the books I was reading, and to my surprise, I was able to make an appointment with every single one I called. Having been in business for 34 years, I knew that most people in the business world are at their desk at 4:30 in the afternoon. That's when I called. I got every single person I wanted to speak to on the line. I got an appointment with Dr. James Forsyth, Suzanne Somers' doctor. I got an appointment with Cancer Treatment Centers of America and several other less notable doctors. I guess in a world with a 98% death rate for stage IV patients within five years, everybody's looking for a new pipeline of patients to replenish the ones that are dying off. Statistically, it would seem every oncologist would have to take every Stage IV patient just to make the payments on the Mercedes.

THE EMAIL FROM JAN

At about the time I received my port, I just quit reading my emails from work. As the CEO of a multimillion-dollar company, I literally had over 1,000 emails a day. It was overwhelming, tedious, and no longer important to me. I couldn't focus on myself, much less be concerned about anything outside of my body. I was just too sick at the time. On top of the weakness from the chemotherapy, the pain from the port just about did me in. I literally did not move my arm for three weeks. I was still losing about a half a pound to a pound a day, and at this point, I had lost a total of about 15 pounds ... and all my hair. I felt like the people really close to me would call or text. I could do everything else when I felt better. This would prove to be a gross error.

STUDYING EVERYTHING ON CANCER

I immersed myself morning, noon, and night reading, studying, and becoming an expert on cancer. I studied every single word in every single text. I cross-referenced everything from my books with my iPad. I noted everything that concerned me and taped it to the wall. I was laboring away full time designing a plan of care and a plan of action to battle this cancer. To lift myself up emotionally, I put up over 50 self-motivation cards with sayings such as, "Pray every day."

To get back to my studies, I would race through my emails, printing them out and setting them aside to read later. My goal was to get off the computer as rapidly as possible so that David could get back to work. We only had one computer.

The day after I had my port surgery was my worst day of pain and suffering. I printed off all my emails and set them on the end table beside the loveseat in the living room. David and I had chosen seats as soon as we walked into the apartment, with him taking the couch and I taking the loveseat. All my documentation was piled on the end table. I continued my research, and every day piled new emails on top of the old ones. It soon grew to quite a stack. I never really seemed to find the time to catch up on my work. I had my research to do and it was all-consuming.

It is startling to wake up one day and realize my life's work—to which I gave my heart and soul, loved every minute of, dreamed, slept, and couldn't wait to get back to—was no longer important when facing the prospect of imminent death. I forgot everything else. While I still loved my employees dearly, my head was no longer in the game. Sales goals were not important. Return on investment was not important. I was the one that always drove them. The things that got me excited before just didn't matter anymore.

My basic personality is to research, strategize, develop a plan, and execute the plan while achieving the goal, and that was moving at 200%. I had to find a way to battle this cancer. I just had no way of knowing that my solution was going to come from one of my employees—Jan—whom I loved dearly.

THE APARTMENT

Chemotherapy came, and chemotherapy went. Week in and week out the days moved by very slowly as I found myself in terrible pain but refused to take any pain medication for fear of further impacting my immune system negatively. I wasn't helping this cancer kill me.

Our apartment was a mess. David and I have always kept an immaculate house. David is a clean freak and I try to humor him to make him happy. We had both been distracted as the apartment was hardly home. It just didn't really make sense to spend any time picking it up. We had a housekeeper that came once a week, so it was not dirty. There was just all my stuff everywhere, taped to the walls, piled up on the coffee table on the end tables, stacked on the floors, and pretty much everywhere else. So, before I left for home, I cleaned everything up and put everything away.

THE NEULASTA LIE

MD Anderson told me that I could go home on August 29, 2012, if I gave myself a Neulasta shot. That way they would not make me stay and I could leave immediately following chemotherapy if I gave myself the medicine on the way home. I gave myself the shot without looking it up, but I wished I had. When I had the time to look it up, I found that it tended to cause the tumors to grow additional blood vessels (angiogenesis). Neulasta causes cancer growth! This drug is designed to boost the bone marrow depression associated with chemotherapy and increase the white count, red count, and platelet count. The price is terrible achy bone pain and increased angiogenesis. It causes cancer to grow! I was horrified!

HOME

It was so nice to come home. While we'd only been gone six weeks, it felt like forever. My last chemotherapy had been a full dose plus 20%, which just about killed me. I had lost so much weight and was so sick, I couldn't think.

Five days at home flew by and it was time to go back to MD Anderson. It's a 10-hour drive to Houston from our home, which gave me plenty of time to read the book *Anticancer*. The best thing about that book was the scientific basis from which the book was written that appealed to my scientific side. I found the footnotes of the book to be extraordinary, particularly an article by Stephen Jay Gould entitled, "The Median is Not the Message." This article discusses how Gould, a statistician, came down with cancer and immediately raced out to look at the survival statistics, which were dismal. Being a statistician, he realized immediately that cancer survival statistics were based on the median, which is the sum of months lived after diagnosis divided by the number of patients in the study. This meant that some patients died immediately, and some lived significantly longer. The goal is to push yourself out to the far end of the tail of the bell-shaped curve. Gould lived 20 years after his diagnosis. I was going to figure out how to live long enough to be considered the far end of the bell-shaped curve.[12]

HOPE

When David and I walked into our apartment, there was a piece of paper laying in the middle of the coffee table. As our living room had been immaculate when we left, I immediately assumed that the landlord has been in and left us a notice. I picked up the notice and it was an email dated August 17, 2012 from my employee Jan Steele, RN. Jan's email told me about an article on PubMed, about a doctor in Vienna, Austria who saved a woman with ovarian cancer by using alkaline therapy, hyperthermia, low dose-dose dense chemotherapy, dendritic cells, nutritional therapy, immunotherapy and IV vitamin C. The doctor's name was Ralf Kleef. I had read a book, The Power of Two, in which the patient received the first dendritic cells in America. I was very interested in dendritic cells as a primary protein building block of the immune system as I didn't see how chemotherapy—which destroyed the immune system—could make me well. It didn't make sense. I knew the immune system had to function for me to survive.

I immediately called Jan. My cell phone was not international, but my office phone is, and I owned the company. Jan called Dr. Kleef and got me an appointment for September 29. I called my son-in-law, who went the next day, and set my cell phone up for international calling. ***I had hope.***

DR. KLEEF

I immediately called Dr. Kleef back, and had a wonderful conversation with him. He developed a treatment plan for me that included finishing my last round of chemotherapy on September 11, 2012, and then flying to Vienna, Austria. Dr. Kleef said, "What is stopping you from beginning your healing journey?" I stammered that my appointment date was September 29, 2012 and that was why I delayed. Dr. Kleef replied, "I will see you whenever you show up." He did. His entire staff came in on a holiday and I was their only patient on September 17, 2012.

Dr. Kleef had come up with a comprehensive plan for wellness that included an initial evaluation of my current post-chemotherapy status. In Europe, medicine is done differently. With your doctor, you select the therapies that you would like from a menu. There are no clinical trials. Dr. Kleef spent his initial time with me boosting my immune system for surgery.

After two weeks of outpatient therapy in Dr. Kleef's clinic, David and I were off October 2, 2012, to Germany for my hysterectomy with an eleven-day hospitalization. There was no cancer found during the operation. Then it was back to Dr. Kleef for three rounds of post-operative chemotherapy with alkaline therapy, hyperthermia, low dose dense chemotherapy, dendritic cells, nutritional therapy, immunotherapy and IV vitamin C.

Dr. Kleef continued my search for natural ways to cure cancer combined with allopathic ways. Without his guidance and treatment, I would not be here. To cure advanced symptoms of metabolic disturbances that appear as cancer takes a comprehensive approach of allopathic medicine, combined with naturopathic, Kinesiology with Muscle Testing, Iridology, Reflexology and Massage, Homeopathy, Aromatherapy, and Bach Flowers remedies.

To cure cancer and to improve my health, I own a Photon Genius which is the only legal hyperthermia machine in the US. I also own a BioCharger, a frequency machine that measures the time it takes an electron to make a complete revolution around a molecule.[13] I own the entire Bob Beck Protocol, an Alternating Current (AC) electricity machine that kills germs, a Direct Current (DC) electricity machine that increases healing, an Ozonator, and a Colloidal Silver machine. I own a foot bath that decreases the toxic burden in the body. I own Kinesiology Chips that have frequency in them. I own an energy cleaner I sleep on every night. I own a Halo machine with multiple alkaline herbal remedies. I own a Rife Machine which also works on frequency. I own a Kangan water machine to create hydrogen rich, alkaline water.

These machines, supplements, good clean water and an improved lifestyle combined with the knowledge I have gained, and my own self-study have allowed me to live.

I wish I could say this was the end of the cancer battle, but it was not. It was just the beginning. This details just the first few months. In the years since, I have tried everything. I have had chemotherapy, surgery, and radiation. I have used all naturopathic modalities. I have had cyberknife and radiation narcosis. This was misdiagnosed as another brain tumor. Through it all, my employees held steadfast. Naturopathic medicine brought me to where I am today. I can work, walk, talk, and remember everything. Julia has TRS Healthcare now, which is the largest, privately held travel nurse agency in the United States. I am able to work.

I have had a hard road. I have turned around, from the chemical medicine of man of the allopathic community of which I was a part for 40 years, to embracing the naturopathic world of God. I don't care what the name of the treatment is, everything must be done to beat the metabolic disturbance known as cancer, as this is a fearsome enemy. I have survived for nine years. There is no cancer.

CHAPTER 2: INTERNAL FORTITUDE: AFTER CANCER OR ADVANCED DISEASE CONTINUE TO FIGHT

"You restored me to health and let me live. Surely it was for my benefit that I suffered such anguish. In your love you kept me from the pit of destruction; you have put all my sins behind your back."
- Isaiah 38:16-17

After the treatment of cancer or advanced disease of any type, the body must be rebuilt. This is hard to do and requires much time. To be successful, you must not give up! Every day, your body is rebuilt a little at a time.

This is a time that requires an "attitude of gratitude." You are still alive! There is much to live for! Coming back after cancer or advanced disease requires a high degree of internal fortitude. It also takes a warfare approach in the face of the limited ability of the medical industry to eradicate cancer or advanced disease while at the same time devastating the body. Chemotherapy, Radiation, and Surgery causes great damage. It takes years to eliminate medical toxins from the body **after** medical treatment.

You must have a strategy and a plan; execute it, and reach deep down into yourself and decide that you really want to be the best you can be. This requires a great deal of Internal Fortitude. An advanced disease-fighting, complementary protocol is not going to be easy. It will take discipline, time management, and lots of prayer. Internal Fortitude is a decision you make every day. Get up every morning and ask yourself if you are doing everything you can to fight, and if not, are you choosing to do things to make disease grow?

Discipline is a state of mind. Becoming disciplined is easy—you decide to do your list of advanced disease or cancer fighting tasks and you just do them. This is self-discipline. Self-discipline is the first step in deciding to have self-control and doing what is **needed** rather than doing what you **want to do. Being disciplined gives you the ability to forego the current momentary desire, for the future benefit of a longer life.**

Next, decide you will do whatever it takes to reach maximum wellness. Decide that you will follow whatever plan might make a difference in giving your body the very best opportunity to get well. Make a covenant with God! You will have to give yourself a shot possibly, drink foul tasting concoctions and devote time and money to getting well. You are your own boss, in charge of your medical treatment and not a mere spectator. You decide how you live.

Time management is critical in any disease-fighting plan as there will be multiple steps that must be combined to create the synergy needed to stop the disease from growing and rebuilding the body. Appointments must be scheduled, meals cooked (these need to be as organic as possible), supplements and nutraceuticals must be taken on schedule, medicines must be taken as needed, exercise scheduled, and all this managed. This is in addition to work, home duties, children, and relatives.

Remember that this schedule will probably have to be followed for at least 1-2 years, some parts for up to 5 years and some things, such as diet and detox, indefinitely. It is a long-term time management project to recover from cancer, or other advanced diseases.

Know that it will have side effects. These side effects could be mental, physical, or emotional. Knowing this in advance makes it easier to deal with when facing hard decisions. It is very easy to feel cheated or jealous of others when you are dealing with so much and they seem to be doing so well. Do not compare yourself to them—just be grateful to be alive. Maybe your challenge is something as simple as everyone you are with is eating ice cream and you have made a decision not to eat sugar.

Handle every day problems with prayer or meditation. Be grateful, this emotion is measured at 500 Hz! To give yourself internal fortitude you have to ask for the grace to make the decisions you have to make, execute the list of actions it takes to control the advanced disease or cancer and then give thanks for the gifts you have received. Always give thanks and praise for your strength. Ask God for wisdom, guidance, and strength. Thank God every day for healing you from this cancer. Visualize yourself as a small child holding out your hands to our Father God and asking for a total and complete healing. Forgive everyone everything. Say: "I forgive everyone, I can, I do, and I will." Prayer increases alkalinity and electrical frequency.

If you feel yourself getting weak, start praying or meditating. It is only through the combined efforts of faith and medicine that the curative effects of medicine can be optimized, and any side effects can be managed.

You must not own the advanced disease or cancer. You must not say "my disease," as it is not yours, even though it has inhabited your body. You must not own this evil Beast! It belongs to Satan, not to you. We cannot allow any negative feelings to overcome our level of effort or progress or our level of commitment.

CHAPTER 3: REBUILDING THE IMMUNE SYSTEM

"And my God will meet all your needs according to the riches of his glory in Christ Jesus." - Philippians 4:19

The cornerstone of rebuilding your body is a strong immune system. This is critical. A strong immune system is the first place to start in preventing disease and successfully rebuilding the body. Without a fully functioning immune system, allergies multiply. These same allergies decrease as the immune system is made stronger.

HOW TO INCREASE THE IMMUNE SYSTEM

1. Vitamin C

Vitamin C inactivates viruses and bacteria while strengthening the immune system. 10,000 mg or 10 Grams by mouth will strengthen the immune system. Linus Pauling studied vitamin C thoroughly and as early as 1940's, he proposed intravenous vitamin C in extremely large doses to kill cancer. This is part of the treatment I had for 5 years.

Vitamin C assists the body in creating glutathione, the strongest antioxidant, and it assists the body in developing Interferon.

The normal dose of oral vitamin C is 6 -10 grams. This creates protection for the body by fighting disease in large quantities of up to 50,000 mg by mouth.

2. Beta Glucans/Mushrooms

Beta Glucans, or a combination of mushrooms, are an immune stimulator that interacts with certain immune cells to activate Galt in the gut. The GALT exists in the intestinal walls and is known to play an important role in healthy immune function.

3. Vitamin D3

Vitamin D3 is known to kill fungi, viruses, bacteria, and parasites. Vitamin D3 over 100 ng/ml is said to prevent cancer growth. A normal blood level is 60-100 ng/ml.

According to Dr. John Cannel, when you get the flu supplement by taking 50,000 IU per day for the first 5 days then drop down to 5,000-10,000IU daily. This was written years before COVID, but it is the recommendation.

I have my vitamin D3 blood level checked every month, then titrate accordingly.

4. Colloidal Silver

Colloidal Silver binds to the DNA of the disease cell, interrupting its reproduction. It also binds with the membrane of the cell, cutting off its oxygen and suffocating it. Silver prevents the transmission from one host to another, thereby preventing person-to-person transmission.

Colloidal Silver can be dosed at 10-20 ppm.

Interestingly, in the Middle Ages, men kept their silver coins in their cod pieces, close to their scrotum. When they camped for the night, they drew a pail of water out of a creek, threw in their silver, waited until morning and the water would be safe to drink, as silver kills fungi, viruses, bacteria, and parasites.

5. Elderberry Tea

Elderberry Tea syrup can be a safe and effective way to boost the immune system.

My Recipe:

Buy dried Elderberries and put two cups in 8 cups of water and boil in the crockpot for two days. Put water in to make eight cups. Skim off the Elderberries. Add three 8-ounce containers of honey, preferably Makuka honey. Add 15 Drops of Copaiba oil, 5 Drops Cinnamon Bark oil plus 1 Teaspoon of dried Cinnamon, 5 Drops Clove Oil, 15 Drops Thieves Oil, 15 Drops Orange Oil, 5 Drops Nutmeg Oil, and 5 Drops Cardamom Oil. Put 3 ounces in the bottom of a coffee cup, top with hot water and enjoy. Or take a tablespoon daily. Refrigerate.

6. Calendula or Melrose Oil

Treats ear infections. Drop 2 to 4 drops into and around ear.

7. Astragulus Root

Astragulus Root has anti-viral properties and boost the immune system

8. Licorice Root
Licorice Root satisfies stomach issues and has strong anti-viral properties, also improving the immune system.

9. Olive Leaf

Olive Leaf kills fungi, viruses, bacteria, and parasites.

10. Adequate Hydration

Correct hydration is drinking ½ of body weight in ounces and add ounces to equal anything that has been drunk. Example: 100 pounds of body weight /.50 = 50 ounces plus 12 ounces for coffee = 62 ounces per day.

11. Sleep 8 hours per day

12. Nasal Irrigation

Nasal Irrigation prior to having nasal drainage. If you are experiencing nasal drainage, do not use. Use Collidial Silver.

13. Zinc

Take 50 mg Zinc as directed, works as an anti-viral and anti-biotic.

14. Echinacea

Take Echinacea as directed, important immunomodulator herb, boosts the immune system.

15. Garlic

Crushed garlic releases allicin, which is a powerful herb that fights fungi, viruses, bacteria, and parasites.

16. Probiotics

Probiotics can be pills or fermented foods. These boost immunity by creating a healthy gut. This may reduce the severity and duration of diseases. Higher colony counts in the colon produce better outcomes in cancer treatments.

THE IMPORTANCE OF DETOXIFICATION (DETOX) CANNOT BE OVEREMPHASIZED

Advanced disease recovery and rebuilding the body after the toxic treatment (chemotherapy, radiation, and surgery) must center on healing the body and the body's image. Our brains hold an image of our bodies—the physical perception of how we look. When the body changes, the brain needs time to catch up. The brain suffers a disconnect when the body does not look like what the brain pictures. This causes grief when that happens, too. The old image is not present anymore. The brain must come to terms with the new body. We must heal physically and emotionally as we rebuild these new bodies.

Anytime a person deals with a diagnosis of cancer or advanced disease, grief and emotional turmoil inevitably begin. My motto has always been, "die before cry," but when I was diagnosed with cancer, I continually cried for a month when faced with my imminent demise. My life was on hold for years as I fought this disease. Treatment, both Allopathic and Naturopathic, meant that my life would never be the same. Often, fighting a diagnosis of cancer or advanced disease is emotionally and physically draining. Many individuals who survive such a diagnosis find they cannot nor do they wish to go back to how life was before their treatment. I was so grateful to be alive! Many find a new normal for them. Things change for them. Some may externally look the same (some do not), but after treatment, different choices are often are made by them for their life. I have had to live with a deformed left breast, multiple surgical scars, brain damage, and many other body image issues. I have had hormonal deficits to contend with. But I chose a new way to live. I was alive! Many call this a "new normal." It took months to recover from cancer and find that "new normal."

Many individuals who survive a diagnosis of cancer or advanced disease find they need time to stop and reflect on what has happened before they can plan for the future. During this process, people may change their values, goals, priorities and outlook on life. It is okay to have "survivor's guilt." Everyone copes with treatment differently. The side effects of treatment can make everyday life difficult.

Rebuilding the body after treatment ends is the key to survival.

Many drugs, especially chemotherapy drugs, are highly toxic at prescribed doses with many side effects. These highly toxic drugs prevent all cells—both malignant and normal—from dividing. This means that many healthy cells in the body are destroyed, leading to adverse chemotherapy long term side effects. Fatigue, brain fog, muscle weakness, neuropathy, loss of energy, malabsorption of nutrients, mood swings, and lack of appetite are all common chemotherapy side effects which remain for years, or even a lifetime, following medical treatment. These treatments are also associated with significant neurotoxicity. Treatments affect both the central and peripheral nervous systems. Biological and immunological therapies have different mechanisms of toxicity. The chemical mix of drug treatments often causes greater physical, psychological, and emotional side effects than the original disease itself. **Detoxifying is essential!**

After chemotherapy or drug treatment, immune system recovery may be slower than expected. The immune system is weakened for up to nine months, especially compromising lung function in vapers and smokers, one study finds. Detoxifying the body from the toxic accumulation of chemicals it has been burdened with during chemotherapy or drugs from advanced disease is essential to recovery.

According to the *American Cancer Society*, more serious and life threatening effects may include renal and liver failure, heart disease, and blood clots, a ill-fated combination of these damaging consequences to the body which often leads to the occurrence of a secondary cancer.

Chemotherapy drugs, their side effects, and the prescribed treatments:

Nitrogen Mustard: The injection site is most susceptible to pain and blood clotting due to this metal-binding chemo compound.

Cisplatin: Known to cause nausea and vomiting starting two hours following treatment. Cisplatin also hinders urination, compromising the removal of toxins. This drug leads to renal (kidney) toxicity.

Doxorubicin: This chemo agent leads to heart damage, including cardiomyopathy (diseased heart) and is a primary trigger for hair loss.

Methotrexate: Known to cause serious, life-threatening side effects such as damage to the lungs, liver, and kidneys. Methotrexate can lower blood cell counts, decreasing the ability to fight infections and interferes with normal blood clotting.

Acyclovir: Prescribed to treat herpes, which is common in patients receiving cytotoxic therapies for cancer. This drug can trigger nausea, vomiting, diarrhea, and decreased urination, which may interfere with the effective removal of toxins. In rare cases, acyclovir can fatally damage the kidneys, resulting in renal failure.

Vincristine: Common effects are bone marrow suppression, gastrointestinal disorder, and neurotoxicity and can lead to renal failure. Infections which typically arise from loss of white blood cells are treated with antibiotics.

Bleomycin: Significantly associated with toxic accumulation in the lungs. Pulmonary toxicity can be life-threatening and progress to lung fibrosis, making it difficult for the lungs to work properly.

Phenothiazines: Relieves symptoms of nausea and vomiting, but causes drowsiness, restlessness, and involuntary movement. These symptoms are then treated with drugs like Benadryl and Cogentin, an anti-tremor medication used in the treatment of Parkinson's disease.

Metoclopramide: Blocks the centers of the brain known as the medulla oblongata to treat nausea. This drug is given to help relieve GI issues and improve blockage of chemicals from intestines. This drug can cause irreversible movement disorders.[14]

Corticosteroids: Synthetic steroids which causes an imbalance in hormones and leads to drowsiness. Generally taken before the start of chemotherapy.

Nabilone: Prescribed for GI complications. Leads to disorientation, low blood pressure, and drowsiness. These symptoms are treated with repetitive rounds of multiple drugs causing mood swings, muscle weakness, easy bruising, and much more.

Detoxification (Detox) means ridding the body of extra toxins from the inside out to improve the immune system, increase fitness and health, and help to heal cancer and other diseases. **To heal, you must have a clean body – so detox.** If cancer patients detox regularly, they will have a clean body. They will experience significantly fewer side effects from cancer cells dying off, a process which releases an endotoxin. Without detoxing, there will be many side effects or symptoms.

Toxins build up in the body from a variety of sources: infections, chemical and environmental pollutants, biotoxins such as fungal, venoms, microbials, plants, or animals. We must rid our bodies of these toxins to prevent side effects up to death.

HERXHEIMER REACTIONS

Herxheimer Reactions, or a cancer die-off reaction, will occur if detoxing is not done and cancer is killed, as it has no way to leave your body. Herxheimer Reactions occur as endotoxins from the death of bacteria, disease, or yeast are released into the body during treatment. These endotoxins are released into the bloodstream and must be eliminated. Detoxing lowers the toxic load that the body must deal with. Since most pollutants and toxins are stored in fat, the best "detox" program pulls the toxins out of the fat reserves. The world we live in continues to have more and more pollutants.

In severe cases, death has occurred if proper detoxing to avoid these symptoms is not implemented. Coffee enemas are known to prevent Herxheimer Reactions.

Common symptoms that develop or worsen due to a Herxheimer response include:

1. Bloating
2. Brain Fog
3. Chills
4. Cold Sweats
5. Constipation
6. Cramps
7. Diarrhea
8. Fatigue
9. Fever
10. Headaches
11. Irritability
12. Joint Pain
13. Lethargy
14. Muscle Pain
15. Nausea
16. Skin Irritation
17. Sore Throat[15]

If you are having any of the symptoms below, start your detox:

1. Fatigued, stress or overwhelmed, always exhausted
2. Headaches and/or lack of mental clarity
3. Skin problems such as skin breakouts, blemishes, and/or a dull complexion
4. Colds, flus, bugs, and viruses

5. On prescription medication
6. Digestion is troublesome, uncomfortable, and irregular
7. Less-healthy food choices, fried foods, processed meat, dairy, gluten, processed foods, refined sugar, or fast food
8. Coffee, alcohol, drugs (prescription or otherwise) or cigarettes
9. Common environmental-toxin exposure such as from carbon emissions, cigarette smoke, herbicides, pesticides, artificial fragrances and household chemicals
10. Excess body weight, struggle to lose weight
11. Feelings are emotionally unstable, depressed, unmotivated, and lacking energy and enthusiasm for life
12. Insatiable sweet tooth
13. Allergies are no longer "seasonal", sinuses drain
14. Joints are sore
15. Just the thought of a detox gives you anxiety
16. Hormones are out of whack
17. Breath and Body odor
18. Sleep patterns are off
19. You are anxious and depressed
20. Cold sores

Rules for Detoxing:

Drink plenty of water, and detox for 30 days if you have cancer or advanced disease.

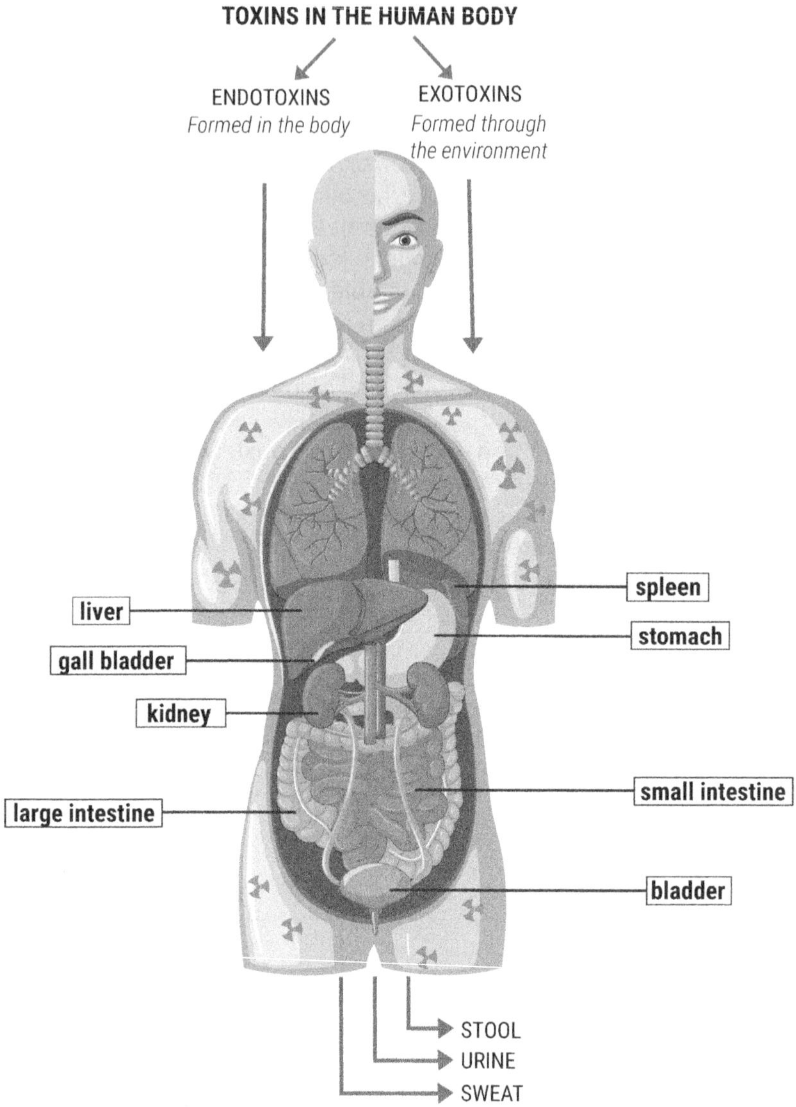

COLON DETOX

Herxheimer Reactions can be reduced, preventing severe reactions or death by ensuring you have a clean colon, and this requires colon cleansing.

COFFEE ENEMAS FOR COLON AND LIVER DETOX:

Wait FOUR HOURS between enemas at a minimum to give your body time to recover.

Ingredients:

1) Use organic coffee only
2) A plastic bucket
3) 5' tubing
4) A red rubber catheter or a enema bag

How to Prepare a Coffee Enema

Combine 3 tablespoons of organic coffee with one quart of distilled, filtered or bottled water. Use a saucepan of at least 1 1/2 quarts.

Bring mixture to a boil. Continue boiling for 3-5 minutes or until the froth has mostly boiled off.

Cover and simmer for 20 minutes. Then filter through a drip-style filter system. Let cool to room temperature.

It seems much easier to use an enema bucket than the enema bags. Fill the bucket (first closing clip around the plastic tubing) to 32 ounces. The bucket or bag should end up about 3 1/2-4 feet from the ground.

Have a timer, a book and music available.

Then use some sort of lubricant on the tip of the catheter you will insert (this is a soft tube and should not hurt at all).

Insert tube and open clip. The coffee will slowly go in as long as you do not have the bucket too high. The higher the bucket, the faster the liquid enters.

Lay on the RIGHT side for this type of enema. Roll onto the knees and forearms to hold it in. Massage the abdomen in a clockwise direction, starting at the lower left and going across and up over the right side, across and then down the left.

Hold it in for 12-15 minutes (that is what the timer is for). Every 3 minutes is a pass thru the liver. It may not be easily done in the beginning, but it is a learned skill. It is usually very relaxing.

Garlic and milk thistle are both good for the colon.

COLON HYDROTHERAPY

High colonics or colonic irrigation are known as colonic hydrotherapy and are used to clean out the colon. This is done by a trained professional.

HERBAL LAXATIVE

1. Psyllium Husk
2. Senna Leaves with fruit
3. Cascara Sagrada
4. Cape Aloe
5. Magnesium

Symptoms that indicate a colon cleanse is needed:

1. Gas and bloating after or between meals
2. Stool
   i. Undigested food particles in stool
   ii. Stool floats in the toilet
   iii. Stringy materials like spaghetti in the stool
   iv. Perfectly uniform round 'things' in the stool
   v. Black flecks in the water of the toilet
   vi. Diarrhea
   vii. Constipation
   viii. Bowel movements fewer than once every day
   ix. Stool doesn't come out quickly
   x. Hemorrhoids
   xi. Pencil thin stools
   xii. Less than 2 bowel movements per day
   xiii. Straining at the stool
   xiv. Stool consistency is not formed (or the consistency of peanut butter)

3. Feels like there's still stool in the rectum after a bowel movement
4. Headaches
5. Stomach pain and Abdominal cramping
6. Nausea
7. Vomiting
8. Depression
9. Anxiety
10. Can't lose weight
11. Poor memory
12. Can't sleep at night
13. Acne
14. Indigestion
15. Allergies
16. Food cravings
17. Sick with colds or flu frequently
18. Hormonal imbalances

19. Body odor
20. Inability to concentrate mentally
21. Fatigue
22. Poor Concentration
23. Bad Breath or Body Odor
24. Sexual dysfunction
25. Appendicitis
26. Rectal fistulas
27. Rectal bleeding[16]

LYMPHATIC DETOX

Lymphatic System helps rid the body of toxins, waste, and other unwanted substances. The lymph is a fluid containing infection-fighting white blood cells throughout the body. The only way the lymph system moves is when the muscles are contracted and expanded.

Signs of a Clogged Lymphatic System:

1. Swelling in hands, feet, and ankles
2. Water retention
3. Muscle and joint stiffness, especially when you first wake up
4. Fibromyalgia
5. Itchy skin
6. Sore throat
7. Fatigue
8. Cellulite[17]

To Cleanse/Drain the Lymphatic System:

1. Bath **Hydrotherapy**, which is a hot-cold shower alternating seven times for 1 minute which contracts and dilates the blood vessels while moving blood which de-congests lymph
2. **Deep breathing** is CRITICAL for pulling toxic waste out because the rib cage is the lymphatic pump.
3. **Walking**
4. **Staying well hydrated**
5. **Increasing potassium intake**, as potassium pulls toxins OUT of the cells. (bananas, oranges, cantaloupe, honeydew, apricots, grapefruit (some dried fruits, such as prunes, raisins, and dates), spinach, broccoli, potatoes, sweet potatoes, mushrooms, peas, and cucumbers)
6. **Consuming an anti-inflammatory alkaline diet** as an alkaline diet including organic fresh produce especially leafy greens and avocados flushes lymph

7. **Eliminating dairy**, which causes the body to produce mucus which increases lymphatic stagnation
8. **Lymph drainage massage**
9. **Raw apple cider vinegar** detoxifies lymph and supports the immune system. I drink ACV Tea for 6 weeks then give my body 2 weeks off. (To make ACV Tea, see page 49)
10. **Limit animal protein and gluten,** as lymph does not drain well in an acidic environment. Too many acidic forming foods are mucus forming, and too much acid waste can damage kidneys. When toxins are not eliminated, they must be stored somewhere, such as the cellulite and the skin
11. **Sweat** is necessary, as the skin is often referred to as the third kidney. Sweating reduces the toxic load on lymph system
12. **Lemons (citrus)** are astringents and cause contraction within lymphatic vessels and nodes helping detoxification
13. **Herbs,** Ex) Ginger and Astragalas
14. **Choose organic fruits and veggies** as toxins in non-organic produce clog lymph. GMOs kill beneficial bacteria in the gut
15. **Do not use antiperspirants;** instead, eliminate dairy, proteins, and medications that cause odor. Or make your own deodorant like I do
16. **Don't shave all the hair off your body,** as hair collects and stores toxins. Skin that is free of hair will cause toxins to irritate the skin which also cause toxins to absorb into the body
17. **Avoid pharmaceutical drugs** as they damage the lymphatic system (always ask your doctor before going off any medication)
18. **Avoid overeating and avoid mixing foods together,** as undigested putrefied food becomes poison and causes lymph stagnation
19. **Negative emotions are toxic and acidic** which clog lymph, so spend time in prayer, forgiveness, meditation, and stress management
20. **Exercise** moves lymph. Use a Rebounder or to force the lymph to move

SKIN DETOX

A skin detox is done by skin dry brushing or infrared sauna. **Dry brushing** removes dead cells from the skin and moves lymph. You begin by brushing the skin in a circular fashion. Brush every part of the body.

Infrared Sauna uses dry heat to induce perspiration, which clears skin, eliminates toxins and moves lymph.

KIDNEY DETOX

Consider a kidney detox if you experience any of these symptoms consistently:

1. Chronic fatigue
2. High blood pressure
3. Loss of appetite
4. Increased or constant urge to urinate
5. Concentration issues
6. Muscle cramps
7. Frequent nausea or vomiting
8. Shortness of breath
9. Swelling of the extremities
10. Chest pain
11. Chronic kidney or UTI infections
12. Trouble sleeping

KIDNEY CLEANSE

Start your day with a cup of hot, Apple Cider Vinegar (ACV) tea before breakfast, as this will allow your system to flush away toxins. Wait two hours to eat.

Apple Cider Vinegar Tea

3 Tablespoons apple cider vinegar (ACV)
10 Drops Lemon Essential Oil (I use Young Living) or Fresh Lemon juice
1 Tablespoon maple syrup ONLY (No sugar, artificial sweeteners, or honey)
¼ teaspoon cayenne pepper
Hot water to fill up the cup

Start slowly, with the daily tea and sip small amounts throughout the day, for those with sensitive stomachs. If the stomach is not sensitive, then you may take the tea at once. Include the drink in your diet to remove the "sand" in your kidneys, so they do not grow into stones.

Cleansing kidneys regularly while living a kidney-supporting lifestyle by using the following is critical to your overall kidney health:

1. Lemon juice
2. Cilantro
3. Dandelion tea
4. Marshmallow root
5. Nettle tea

6. Parsley
7. Red clover
8. Ginger
9. Turmeric
10. Watermelon
11. Pumpkin seeds
12. Blackcurrant juice
13. Cranberry juice
14. Grapes
15. Spirulina
16. Blueberries
17. Millet
18. Barley
19. Asparagus
20. Baking soda (prevents decline of kidney function)

LIVER CLEANSE

Liver cleanses usually rely on apples. According to Richard Gerhauser, MD, apples should never be eaten due to the fact that Canadian scientists' genetically-modified apples to never have brown spots and have a resistance to kanamycin, an antibiotic. The enzyme that is disabled is the one that causes brown spots. The plan was to use these apples for baby food. Under current law, GMOs never need safety testing.[18]

Frequently a liver cleanse may be necessary if you have any of the following problems:

1. History of alcohol/drug use or hepatitis
2. Long-term prescription drug use
3. Sensitivity to chemicals (tobacco smoke, fumes, perfume, cleaning agents, etc.)
4. Pain between the shoulder blades
5. Stomach upset by greasy foods
6. Greasy or shiny stools
7. History of nausea, motion sickness, or morning sickness
8. Pale stools
9. Headache over the eyes
10. Gallbladder attacks
11. Bitter taste in the mouth (especially after meals)
12. Become sick or easily intoxicated if drinking wine
13. Easily hung over
14. Pain under right side of rib cage
15. Hemorrhoids or varicose veins
16. NutraSweet (aspartame) consumption

17. Chronic fatigue
18. Fibromyalgia
19. Acne
20. Frequent alcohol consumption
21. Drank too heavily on a night out or over the weekend
22. Eat processed foods often
23. Sugar intake is moderate to high
24. Feel fatigued, run down, or just tired throughout the day
25. Use chemicals to clean your home
26. Exposed to environmental toxins and pollution (maybe you live in a large city or your workplace uses chemicals)
27. Blood sugar fluctuates often (due to your liver's overburdened state)
28. Skin is always dry
29. Use skincare and cosmetics that contain chemicals daily like lotions, shampoos, conditioners, foundation, etc.
30. Unexplained back pain
31. High Blood Pressure

DR. AXE'S 6-STEP LIVER CLEANSE[19]

Follow these six steps to help boost your health and vitality:

1. Remove Toxic Foods from Your Diet

If you are eating a diet high in processed foods, you are putting the health of your liver at risk, as these foods basically work against liver health. Hydrogenated oils, refined sugar, convenience foods and lunch meats are notoriously toxic to your system.

Hydrogenated oils, also known as "trans fats," have higher levels of saturated fat. The chemical structure of the oil itself has been altered to increase shelf life. Consumption of trans fats dramatically increases the risk for heart disease by 25 percent or more. In addition, it is believed that trans fats cause problems with our immune system and can lead to inflammation throughout the body.

Added nitrates, commonly found in convenience foods, fast foods and lunch meats, have been linked to serious health conditions. These chemicals are used to preserve foods to make them last longer, inhibit bacteria growth and preserve color. Replace these foods immediately with liver- friendly healthful choices. Healthful foods taste great, and, with a bit of creativity, you can create healthful meals for your family that will support liver health.

Roast your own organic chicken breast and turkey breast to replace deli meats for quick lunches and after-school snacks. Replace chips and other processed snacks with fresh fruit, carrot sticks, nuts, and homemade granola bars.

In addition to having a healthful diet, it's important that your digestive enzymes are functioning properly. Problems with liver enzymes can also contribute to liver disease and may be related to other digestive illnesses such as Crohn's disease.

2. Drink Raw Vegetable Juice

It is nearly impossible to eat all of the raw vegetables you need to effectively cleanse your liver. However, by juicing a variety of raw vegetables, you can easily get the 4–5 servings of fresh, organic vegetables you need. Even vegetables that aren't your favorites can be disguised and enjoyed in a fresh vegetable juice!

With impaired liver function, juicing vegetables has the added benefit of making the vegetables easier to digest and more readily available for absorption.

Vegetables ideal for liver cleanses include cabbage, cauliflower, and Brussels sprouts. While that combination may not sound too palatable, you can add other vegetables to the mix that you enjoy, including carrots, cucumber, beets and greens.

All of these vegetables help to reduce acid levels in the body, helping to create a more friendly pH balance. Experiment with your favorite flavor combinations; you can add fresh herbs, including parsley and mint to make the juices more enjoyable.

Fresh, organic carrots are essential to any liver cleanse. In the liver, the beta carotene is converted into vitamin A to help flush out the toxins in the body while reducing fat in the liver.

The high-fiber content helps support a healthy digestive tract, hastening the elimination of toxins in your body. The ginger root helps to soothe the digestive tract, reduce intestinal gas, and has strong anti-inflammatory compounds. The fresh oranges in this recipe not only add tangy sweetness, but also add significant vitamin C, additional vitamin A and vitamin B6.

3. Load Up on Potassium-Rich Foods

Are you getting the recommended 4,700 milligrams per day of potassium?

Chances are, you aren't. Potassium-rich foods help to lower systolic blood pressure, lower cholesterol and support a healthy cardiovascular system, in addition to helping cleanse your liver.

→ Sweet Potatoes

A single medium-sized sweet potato contains nearly 700 milligrams of potassium, not to mention the high fiber and beta carotene content. A sweet potato has more potassium than a banana.

A sweet potato only has 131 calories, yet is rich with vitamins B6, C, D, magnesium, and iron. While naturally sweet, the sugars actually are slowly released into the bloodstream through the liver, without causing a spike in blood sugar.

→ Tomato Sauces

Potassium, and the other beneficial nutrients in tomatoes, is significantly concentrated as a sauce, puree or as a paste. As an example, one cup of tomato puree contains 1,065 milligrams of potassium, but one cup of fresh tomatoes contains only 400 milligrams. When selecting tomato sauce, paste or puree, be sure to choose those made only from organic tomatoes.

To make your own concentrated tomato sauce, slice organic tomatoes in half and roast face down in the oven for 30 minutes at 425 degrees F, until the skin has shriveled. Remove from the oven, and let cool. Slide the skins off and gently crush in your food processor or blender. Strain to remove seeds, if desired. Pour into a Dutch oven, and let simmer until thick, 1-2 hours.

→ Beet Greens and Spinach

Rich in antioxidants, beet greens contain over 1,300 milligrams of potassium per cup. Add beets and beet greens to your fresh vegetable juice recipe; finely chop and add raw to salads; or sauté lightly, like other greens. Beets also naturally cleanse the gallbladder and improve bile flow.

Fresh organic spinach is easily added to your diet, and it's a good source of potassium, containing 840 milligrams per serving.

→ Beans

White beans, kidney beans and lima beans are all rich in potassium, protein, and fiber. Swap out garbanzo beans for one of these potassium-rich beans in your favorite hummus recipe. Enjoy it with carrot sticks and celery sticks.

→ Blackstrap Molasses

Just two teaspoons of this rich, all-natural syrup contains ten percent of the daily-recommended amount of potassium. In addition to potassium, blackstrap molasses is rich with iron, calcium, manganese and copper.

Incorporate blackstrap molasses into your diet by using it to replace other natural sweeteners. You can use it to create barbecue sauces and to top oatmeal or quinoa porridge in the mornings. Two teaspoons added to coffee intensifies the richness of the coffee, while lowering the acidic taste.

→ Bananas

And finally, add a banana to your favorite smoothie. While in comparison to the other high potassium foods on this list, the banana's 470 milligrams of potassium are only part of the story. Bananas assist in digestion, and help to release toxins and heavy metals from the body – all of which are essential during a liver cleanse.

Please note: If you have high levels of potassium in your kidneys, foods rich in potassium should be consumed moderately.

4. Take Milk Thistle, Dandelion and Turmeric Supplements

→ Milk Thistle

Milk thistle is considered the "king" of detoxifying herbs, making it ideal for a liver cleanse. Milk thistle helps to eliminate the buildup of heavy metals, prescription medications, environmental pollutants and alcohol in the liver.

In addition, it helps to reduce the negative effects on the liver after chemotherapy and radiation. The active ingredient, silymarin, helps to strengthen the cell walls in the liver, while supporting healthy regeneration.

Milk thistle can be taken as a supplement or as a liver cleansing detox tea.

→ Turmeric

Turmeric reduces joint pain; is an effective antidepressant; aids in digestion; helps to restore a healthy blood sugar balance; and supports healthy liver tissue and liver metabolism.

Currently, researchers are studying turmeric for a variety of health benefits for diseases and conditions, including: Alzheimer's disease, cancer, depression, osteoarthritis, breast health, prostate health and chronic pain.

→ Dandelion Root

Most homeowners hate the dandelion, as it populates yards every spring, but this flower, and its root, is actually packed with vitamins and minerals.

Dandelion root has a natural diuretic effect, allowing your liver to eliminate toxins more quickly. It also helps to strengthen the immune system, balance blood sugar levels, relieve heartburn, and soothe digestive upset.

Burdock root is another option in the same plant family as dandelions that can help detox your system by cleansing the blood, therefore helping to support liver function. Like milk thistle, both dandelion root and burdock root can be taken in both supplement form or as a detox tea.

5. Eat Real Liver or Take Liver Tablets

Liver from young, healthy, grass-fed cattle or chicken liver is rich in vitamins A and B, folic acid, choline, iron, copper, zinc, chromium and CoQ10. Liver is one of the most nutrient-dense foods we can eat.

If you can't stomach eating liver, you can take beef liver pills. Seek a supplement that guarantees no hormones, pesticides or antibiotics are used in the feeding and care of the cattle.

A QUICK-START 24-HOUR LIVER CLEANSE

In addition to the healthful foods and supplements mentioned above, you can give your liver a boost by starting with a quick, 24-hour liver cleanse. In the seven days prior to this short cleanse, eat kale, cabbage, lettuce, cauliflower, broccoli, Brussels sprouts, citrus fruits, asparagus, beets, and celery. Avoid any processed foods, and eat free-range organic meats, and only sparingly eat gluten and refined carbohydrates. This preparation will help facilitate the cleanse.

During the week you are preparing your body, try Diana's AVC Tea. It boosts your energy and helps you to detox and cleanse the liver.

Then, during the week of your cleanse, try this liver detox drink, which will help support your body while cleansing:

LIVER DETOX DRINK

1. Dilute cranberry juice with a ratio of 3 parts water to 1 part cranberry juice.
2. Add 1/4 teaspoon each of nutmeg and ginger and a 1/2 teaspoon of cinnamon into a tea infuser and let steep in simmering water for 20 minutes.
3. Allow to cool to room temperature.
4. Add the juice of 3 oranges and 3 lemons and stir. If the mixture is too tart, sweeten with your favorite all-natural sweetener.
5. Sip throughout the day.

You should consume a minimum of 72 ounces of this mixture and 72 ounces of water. After one day of the cranberry juice blend, reintroduce the foods you ate in preparation for the liver cleanse.

Final Thoughts

- Cleansing and detoxing the liver and colon helps to clear pesticides, medications, heavy metals, and the remnants of cancer therapy out of your system, resulting in a healthy liver.
- To keep your liver healthy through the years, periodically do a 24-hour liver cleanse.
- Maintain a healthful diet void of processed foods and high in vegetables, legumes and whole grains, whether on a liver cleanse or not.

The 6-Step Liver Cleanse

1. Remove toxic foods from your diet.
2. Drink raw vegetable juice.
3. Load up on potassium-rich foods.
4. Do a coffee enema.
5. Take milk thistle, dandelion and turmeric supplements.
6. Eat liver or take beef liver tablets for maximum B Vitamins.

These herbs will stimulate, tone, and rebuild your liver so that it can release the stored-up toxins from the chemical drugs. These herbs can be taken as a tea or in capsule form:

- Dandelion Root
- Oregon Grape Root
- Turkey Rhubarb Root
- Yellowdock Root[20]

PARASITE CLEANSE

Needed annually.
Symptoms of intestinal parasites:

1. Digestive problems, including unexplained constipation, diarrhea, or persistent gas
2. Skin problems, including unexplained rashes, eczema, or hives
3. Muscle and joint pain
4. Fatigue
5. Lack of satiation after meals
6. Constant hunger
7. Teeth grinding during sleep
8. Anxiety
9. Itchy skin
10. Yeast infections
11. Loss of appetite
12. Iron deficiency
13. Itching of the anus or vagina[21]

Other Symptoms indicating a Parasite Cleanse is needed:

1.Crawling Sensations

If parasites are located close to the skin or within the digestive tract, you may be able to feel them. Additionally, it is possible to feel parasites moving around the tongue, throat, and cheek areas of the face.

2. Headaches and Pain

Headaches and pain throughout the body are a common symptom of Lyme and parasite die-off. Headaches can also be a result of parasites moving around inside the head. In these circumstances, pain may be located behind or inside of the eyes, around the ears, or all over. Hot baths and gentle massaging can assist in reducing the pain.

3. Fatigue and Weakness

When you consider the fact that parasites like Giardia can be responsible for causing chronic fatigue syndrome, it's easier to accept that you might feel some fatigue temporarily during the process of eliminating parasites from your system. It's worth noting that it takes a great deal of energy for your body to rid itself of parasites. Once most of the Lyme or parasites in your system have been eliminated, you will begin to regain your energy and strength. However, to speed the healing process, it may be best to avoid excessive activity and exercise and get plenty of sleep.

4. Skin Sores

Skin sores are yet another common symptom of die-off. These sores can occur when the body tries to eliminate toxins at a quicker pace than is generally possible. The skin is one of the organs that can be used to get rid of toxins, and if too many toxins attempt to leave the skin at once, this can lead to breakages and sores. Toxins that leave the body by breaking through the skin might include eggs, parasite waste, or the parasites themselves.

5. Digestive Problems

Digestive problems are issues that can start to arise when the parasite is still living within your body, but in some cases, these issues may appear to get worse when you begin your parasite or Lyme cleanse. Depending on the severity of the parasite you are trying to remove, you could experience instances of bloating and diarrhea. Some people feel strange knots or lumps develop around the belly button, too.

6. Emotional Instability

Parasites survive by consuming the nutrients that you need to thrive. The result of such deficiencies is often periods of anxiety, depression, and confusion. Additionally, the other symptoms that you are exposed to during die-off can lead to heightened emotions, as well. The best thing to do in this situation is look around for support and remember that you need to go through the negative stages in order to remove the parasite or Lyme from your body entirely. After all, you don't want to live with a parasite, or chronic Lyme disease forever.

7. Easy or More Frequent Bruising

The result of this parasite restlessness means that you will begin to feel the creatures moving around inside of your body – potentially looking for a new place to live. Whatever the reason for the movement, when parasites move too close to the skin, the result can be easier bruising. You might find yourself covered in bruises, even if there is no apparent reason.

8. Cravings

Parasites and Lyme disease feed on specific foods within your body more readily than others. For instance, the most important thing you will do when conducting a Lyme disease cleanse is to remove grains and sugars from your diet. It's also a good idea to avoid animal-based foods because they can slow down digestion and make it harder for the body to eliminate parasites. Because you will be cutting certain foods out of your diet – specifically the ones that your parasites prefer—it's common to feel cravings during the first few days as your body adjusts. Make sure that you don't give into these cravings, if you want the cleanse to work.

9. Respiratory Effects

Finally, the destruction of parasites may cause your body to take drastic measures to remove the foreign invaders as quickly as possible. Since increasing the flow of mucous is often seen as an effective way to rid the body of other contaminants, the chances are that you will experience several respiratory symptoms like those of the common cold, including sneezing, coughing, and a runny or stuffy nose.

Natural herbs that possess powerful anti-parasitic properties include:

1. Wormwood
2. Oregano oil
3. Black walnut
4. Berberine
5. Grapefruit seed extract
6. Papaya seed
7. Pumpkin seed
8. Garlic

One Parasite Cleanse that works is Paratrex, another is Fenbenzadole when used as directed. Paratrex smells wonderful, like your grandmother's spice cabinet. Fenbenzadole FOR 10 pounds dog is tasteless and odorless.

PETROCHEMICAL WEIGHT LOSS DETOX

This detox removes harmful petrochemicals that are stored in the fat of the body. You can expect to see cellulite smooth out and a loss of several inches, with a weight loss of several pounds. The petrochemicals must be removed for weight loss to occur.

Three-Week Protocol

You will need:

- 3 bottles of Citrus Fresh essential oil blend by Young Living
- 1 bottle of Juva Cleanse essential oil blend by Young Living

- 2 bottles of Grapefruit essential oil by Young Living
- 1 Bag of empty vegetable capsules

Instructions

- Mix the 3 bottles of Citrus Fresh with the bottle of Juva Cleanse together in a small glass container with a lid.
- Leave overnight.
- Pour the contents of the glass container back into the 3 bottles of citrus fresh.
- Use 1 bottle of this mixture per week.
- Apply this generously to your target areas. One bottle should be enough for 2 target areas (e.g. stomach and hips). If you have more target areas, you will need more. Do not dilute the oils or it may not work.
- Take 5-12 drops of grapefruit, either internally by using a capsule (available at Young Living) or rubbing this on the target areas also.

Warning: Grapefruit can react to certain medications. Please check your medications before beginning this protocol.

Another thing to note is that citrus essential oils are photosensitive, which means you shouldn't expose your target areas to the sun within 12 hours of applying these oils to the skin.

You may also experience detox symptoms from this protocol while the toxins are being removed from your body.[22]

IONIZING FOOTBATH

An ionic foot detox works by pulling the toxins out of your body through your feet. The ionizing machine works to ionize the foot bath water with an array. This process is said to give the hydrogen in the water a positive charge which pulls out toxins from the feet.[23]

This ionic foot detox decreases the inflammation in the body.

To decrease inflammation: The foot bath is run repeatedly four times, with the water poured down the drain after each ionic foot detox. The inflammation number can be recorded prior to the ionic foot detoxes and afterward, to show how much the inflammation number has decreased.

CHAPTER 4: POTENTIAL SIDE EFFECTS OF CANCER AND ADVANCED TREATMENT

There are Limited or No Symptoms or Side Effects of Naturopathic Treatment

"My flesh and my heart may fail, but God is the strength of my heart and my portion forever." - Psalms 73:26

The Collateral Damage after Cancer and advanced disease Treatment[24] occurs when healthy tissue is affected when the tumor is treated. Problems occur when tumor growth crowds or invades normal cells. Surgeons require "clear margins" with no evidence of tumor or disease growth, so healthy tissue around a tumor is removed during surgery which may cause side effects. Some side effects occur years after treatment. There are many physical side effects and changes which have emotional components. Body image is one of these.

Medical experts can't always predict if or when side effects will occur, which may be at the time of treatment or even years afterward. These vary, as they can be very mild to serious, and are different, depending on the individual. Some side effects are lasting such as scarring, and some vanish in time. In most cases, the side effects could not have been avoided.[25] Remember that after chemotherapy, surgery, radiation, and advanced disease, there are always side effects. No one gets out of a serious disease unscathed, mentally or physically.

Surgery Side Effects that can occur years later:

- Scarring
- Problems fighting infection

- Lymphedema or swelling of arms or legs
- Nutritional and digestion problems
- Cognitive problems such as trouble focusing or memory loss
- Changes in sexual function or fertility
- Pain that may be chronic or long-term
- Difficulty with speech or swallowing

Chemotherapy Side Effects that can occur years later:

- Fatigue
- Difficulty with focused thinking (sometimes called chemo brain)
- Early menopause
- Heart problems
- Reduced lung capacity
- Kidney and urinary problems
- Nerve problems such as numbness and tingling
- Bone and joint problems
- Muscle weakness
- Secondary cancers

Radiation Therapy Side Effects that can occur years later:

- Cataracts
- Fatigue
- Dry mouth
- Permanent hair loss
- Problems with thyroid or adrenal glands
- Infertility
- Slowed or halted bone growth in children
- Decreased range of motion in the treated area
- Skin sensitivity to sun exposure
- Problems with memory or ability to learn
- Secondary cancers such as skin cancer

Late effects of treatment can affect day-to-day life activities, such as:

- Difficulty working due to physical or emotional issues
- Changes in relationships with loved ones, friends, or coworkers
- Impact on self-esteem
- Difficulty getting health or life insurance
- Difficulty communicating concerns to others
- Financial stress

FATIGUE

Fatigue can be caused by medicines you are taking, pain, and other medical problems that may affect your energy level. Fatigue can be seen as chronic lower body weakness; tightening of the pelvic muscles and vaginismus, a spasmodic contraction of the vagina with pain.

Fatigue can be treated by:

1. Exercise, such as walking
2. Meditation or Relaxation Sessions
3. Changing your diet to the Immune Strengthening Diet[26]
4. Increasing water (drink half your weight in ounces of water and add any number of ounces for everything else you may drink)
5. Nutritional supplements that can help, such as Barley Life, Complete Energy by Nutri-West, NMN, Apple Cider Vinegar, and detoxing
6. Ozone Therapy IV

Limiting Fatigue

1. Plan your day. When a plan is decided on, it gets done!
2. Be aware of when you feel most energetic and active. Plan activities at that time.
3. Changing how you do things to save energy. Sit down to towel off, sit on a stool while you cook or wash dishes. Lean against the washer and dryer when washing clothes.
4. Take short naps or rest breaks daily.
5. Try to go to sleep and wake up at the same time every day.
6. Focus on what you enjoy. Do old or new interests that do not tire you out. Do fewer of all activities.
7. Let others help you. If no one offers, ask for what you need.
8. Just say "no" to things that are not important. Use your energy to live a fuller life.
9. Think about joining a support/education group for people with cancer or other advanced disease. Talking about fatigue with others can teach new ways to cope.

Herbs To fight Fatigue: Look for herbs in tea, liquid, or supplement form.

1. Dehydration – a lack of adequate water in your system causes fatigue.
2. Eat nuts – almonds or peanuts are high in magnesium and folate (folic acid). These nutrients are essential for energy and

cell production. A lack of these nutrients in your system can leave you feeling fatigued. They also produce good fat.

3. Cinnamon oil or stick – a smell of this spice can reduce fatigue.[27]
4. Peppermint Oils - scent is a fatigue fighter.
5. Licorice Root – reduces adrenal fatigue which you likely have after dealing with cancer or advanced disease.
6. Panax ginseng - a dietary supplement to improve general well-being, cardiovascular disorders, depression, erectile dysfunction, menopausal hot flashes – and fatigue. If you take antidepressants, diabetes, or blood-thinningmedications, consult your physician first.
7. Maca - a caffeine-like energy driver, less the jitters and shakes. People who use maca root continuously report feeling more alert, driven, and energetic. Maca also affects sexual libido.
8. Royal Jelly - milky-white potassium filled substance produced in the glands of nurse bees is widely used for fatigue, depression, and many more ailments. Loaded with B vitamins, Royal Jelly can decrease fatigue and increase endurance by increasing oxygen consumption. Consult with your physician first if you take blood thinners.
9. Siberian Ginsing – (Eleuthero, not a true ginseng) - improves athletic performance, energy, and physical stamina, and focus, and helps manage stress. It improves immune function and hormones, according to Jaquel Patterson, ND, a naturopathic physician.
10. Cordyceps – a medicinal mushroom, improving muscle weakness, and increasing athletic performance, helps combat fatigue with anti-aging and anti-tumorigenic properties and fights inflammation, which may be the cause of fatigue, according to Dr. Patterson.

PAIN

Pain may occur after treatment or be caused by the treatment. Pain is a message sent to the brain that some area of the body is in trouble and needs your attention which is important as it prevents further injury. Pain is counterintuitive—instead of developing a tolerance to pain, it wears down resistance. So, the more pain you experience the less it is tolerated. Decreasing pain allows the client to feel better and stay active.

The types of pain felt following cancer or advanced disease treatment medical treatment may include:

1. Radiation causes skin sensitivity where you received radiation is

a common side effect and can last for many months to years.

2. Neuropathy is pain or numbness in the hands and feet due to injured nerves. Chemotherapy or surgery can damage nerves which can cause severe pain.
3. Surgery (especially on the central meridian on the midline in front or back) can cause painful scars from cancer surgery or advanced disease.
4. Surgical Amputation causes phantom pain in a missing limb or breast. While doctors do not know why this phantom pain occurs, Naturopaths do. It is real because your body still retains the electrical frequency energy of the amputated body part and the body does not know that the amputated part is missing.

Limiting Pain:

1. Lavender essential oil is used to relieve pain, to help with sleep, and to ease anxiety, as well as anti-inflammatory and antioxidant effects.
2. Rosemary essential oil may relieve pain from headaches, muscles and bones, reduce seizures and inflammation, relax smooth muscles, and boost memory.
3. Peppermint essential oil (*Mentha piperita* L. plant) is anti-inflammatory, antimicrobial, and pain-relieving.
4. Eucalyptus essential oil may help reduce pain, swelling, and inflammation in the body.
5. Cloves Oil (*Eugenia caryophyllata* plant) is used to relieve pain from toothache, could relieve other sorts of pain.
6. Capsaicin present in chili peppers, provides natural pain relief by working on nerves that carry pain signals.
8. Ginger (*Zingiber officinale*) may accelerate recovery and reduce inflammation after exercise, a natural pain reliever.
9. Feverfew (featherfew or bachelor's buttons) eases fever, migraine headaches, rheumatoid arthritis, toothaches, and stomach aches, as well as increasing breast milk, reduce inflammation and muscle spasms.
   Talk to your doctor as Feverfew can cause abdominal pain, nausea, vomiting, and increased risk of bleeding.
10. Turmeric or Curcumin (the spice turmeric) has pain-relieving qualities, reducing inflammation. I drink Turmeric every day in my coffee, try adding it to curries, smoothies, or juices, or any dish you cook.
11. Acupressure or massage restores the natural energy flow that flows along the meridians. Heat and cold therapy—apply packs to area that is painful. Experimentation is the best way to find if this is effective.

12. Acupuncture helps reduce chronic pain, low back pain, neck pain, osteoarthritis or knee pain, reduces tension headaches and prevent migraine headaches.
13. Deep Breathing Exercise creates oxygen which is needed for cellular respiration, cellular metabolism, and brain function. Correct breathing is deep abdominal breathing not the shallow breathing into the lungs. Breathe deeply into the abdomen and hold for 7 seconds, to release place the tongue to the roof of the mouth by the teeth and slowly breathe out.
14. Yoga helps manage pain naturally, especially back and neck pain, stress or anxiety. It incorporates stretching, breathing exercises, self-care, and relaxation methods,
15. Mindfulness meditation or biofeedback may teach how to manage chronic pain, pain symptoms, depression, and quality of life.
16. CBD Oil is highly effective for pain, to keep pain under control, do not wait until you hurt to take these medicines. Take as directed.
17. Physical therapy helps by using heat, cold, massage, pressure, and/or exercise to help decrease pain.
18. Braces limits movement of a painful limb or joint.
19. Practicing deep relaxation to help relieve pain or reduced stress.
20. Nerve blocks or surgery often help if you have persistent, limiting pain, but they may put present other problems.

How to write down pain to track changes over time.

a. Describe the pain as sharp, dull, throbbing, steady.
b. Show the exact places it hurts, whether the pain stays in one place or whether it moves around.
c. Use a scale from 0 to 10 with 0 being no pain and 10 being the worst pain you could have.
d. Explain the pain: its duration, strength at various times of day or night, and if anything makes it better or worse.
e. Describe how pain affects your daily life.
f. Talk about any side effects you've experienced with pain-control.

LYMPHEDEMA: ARM OR LEG SWELLING (DETOX!)

Lymphedema is a swelling that is caused by the buildup of lymph fluid in a dependent part of the body, usually an arm or leg. The lymph system is part of the immune system and cannot function properly if it is clogged, so detox! Lymphedema is a side effect for breast cancer, melanoma of the arms and legs, prostate cancer, cancer of female or male reproductive organs, or other lower abdominal-area cancers that have spread. Any time that surgery or radiation therapy is used, and especially after lymph-node removal, there is a higher risk of lymphedema. It can be quite painful. The usual causes are surgery, cancer or the treatment of cancer, or advanced disease.

Signs of Lymphedema:

1. Watch for signs of swelling or infection which are redness, pain, heat, fever. Report these.
2. Keep the arm or leg free of cuts, insect bites, or sunburn.
3. Do not have shots or blood tests done in areas of lymphedema.
4. Eat a well-balanced, protein-rich, low-salt diet.
5. Wear loose-fitting clothing on arms or legs.
6. Do not use that arm or leg to test heat or cold. The swelling may be less capable of feeling differences in temperature.

Treatment for lymphedema consists of relieving the lymphatic system of the burden of draining fluid back out, therefore, increasing venous blood flow should decrease the accumulation of lymph in the connective tissues.

1. Elevation try to keep arm or leg above chest level.
2. Manual Lymphatic Drainage use a professional lymphatic massage certified practitioner trained in this method. This can be very effective with regular use.
3. Self-Lymphedema Massage is long, deep strokes up the affected area. To make a massage oil designed for lymph drainage, use pure essential oils: 6 drops lemongrass, 6 drops grapefruit, 3 drops rosemary, 2 drops tangerine and 2 drops cypress or juniper in 2 ounces of carrier oil.
4. Special bandages and clothing that can help lymph fluid drain.
5. Maintain correct body weight.
6. Yoga increases circulation to move the congested lymph and accumulating fluid.
7. Keep your skin moist and clean; use lotions.
8. Compression stockings to decrease swelling.
9. Diet foods rich in flavonoids such as berries, onions, and citrus fruits which strengthen lymph fluid.
10. Supplements that should be taken are ginkgo, bilberry (*Vaccinium myrtillus*), elderberry (*Sambucus nigra*), vitamin C at least 10-20 Grams per day to bowel tolerance.

Ginkgo, as directed, increases arterial blood flow. It may be more effective with gotu kola (*Centella asiatica*) or horse chestnut seed (*Aesculus hippocastanum*), which are specific for venous insufficiency. Orally taken: The dose of gotu kola is 2-4 grams daily of the dried leaves, or 60-120 mg daily of an extract, standardized to 40% asiaticoside. Gotu kola increases blood flow through the veins by enhancing the surrounding connective tissue.

Orally taken: (*Galium aparine*) A typical formula to move lymph is equal parts of cleavers, mullein (*Verbascum* spp.), prickly ash bark (*Zanthoxylum* spp.) and red clover flowers (*Trifolium pratense*).

ORAL MUCOSITIS OR MOUTH SORES

Damage to the cells in your mouth by treatment can lead to sores and infections which are difficult to heal by themselves. Sores that appear are burn-like and are painful that manifest on soft tissues of the mouth, lips, gums, tongue, roof or floor of the mouth and down the esophagus. The pain from these mouth sores make it difficult to eat, talk, swallow and breathe. The severity of mouth sores can range from minor to a severe complication that may make it difficult to impossible to continue cancer treatment. Treating mouth sores involves decreasing pain until the cells of the mouth heal and begin regenerating.

Cancer treatments, chemotherapy and radiation, work by killing rapidly dividing and growing cells. Healthy cells also divide and grow rapidly, such as hair cells (baldness), or the lining inside the mouth and esophagus. Both chemotherapy and radiation impair the immune system, which allow viruses, bacteria and fungi to infect the mouth and body, causing mouth sores or making mouth sores worse.[28]

Tips for Mouth Sores:

1. Try coating agents with topical painkillers. These medications can be applied directly to mouth sores. Try rinsing the mouth with a mixture of Milk of Magnesia and Lidocaine. A pharmacist can mix this.
2. Change the pH of the mouth; mix a combination of baking soda and warm water solution to swish around in the mouth.
3. Keep mouth moist with water or ice chips, chew sugarless gum or suck on sugar-free hard candy (Remember: Sugar allows cancer to grow. Use a mouth-moistening agent to moisten your mouth.
4. CBD Oil may help to heal these and decrease pain. Hold dropperful in mouth as long as possible, swishing, then swallow.
5. Use a straw while drinking.
6. Toothpaste and mouthwash are natural oral care products that offer anti-inflammatory, antimicrobial, antibacterial and antifungal properties. All of which are advantageous during

chemotherapy. Foam swabs may be preferable to toothbrushes. Floss every day.

7. Stay away from all tobacco products. Stop smoking.
8. Eat a diet rich in fruits and vegetables, avoid meat and acidic or spicy foods that irritate the mouth. Avoid sharp and crunchy foods (chips, crackers and pretzels). Eat small meals more frequently and slowly, while cutting food into small pieces.
9. Alcohol can burn open mouth wounds.
10. Cold therapy (cryotherapy) helps to swish ice chips or cold water around in your mouth for the first half-hour of treatments. The cold limits the amount of the drug that reaches your mouth, reducing your risk of mouth sores.

Some Therapies that may cause Mouth Sores:

1. Head or neck radiation therapy
2. Bone marrow transplant
3. Herpes simplex virus

Severe Complications may require medical intervention:

1. Infection in a weakened immune system. Germs can invade the body causing a massive infection.
2. Chemotherapy reduces your blood's ability to clot, which can mouth sores to bleed; continue rinsing with water. Severe bleeding may require medical assistance.

A HEALTHFUL DIET, AT A HEALTHFUL WEIGHT, WITH A HEALTHFUL LIFESTYLE IS BEST WHEN DEALING WITH WEIGHT CHANGES

Weight loss-or-gain ideas are patient specific, and there is no meal plan that's right for everyone. It's critical to make sure that body weight is at a healthful weight range. Weight may change with increases because you are under stress, on steroids, or certain medications, or it may decrease because of stress, or certain diet.

Side effects from treatments such as chemotherapy, radiation, and surgery or advanced disease can affect appetite, eating habits, activity levels, and weight. Research shows that some cancer survivors who have had certain kinds of chemotherapy or who have taken certain medicines, especially hormone treatments for hormone-driven malignancies such as breast and prostate cancers, may have problems with weight gain. This weight gain affects the chance of recovery. If you're overweight aim for controlled weight loss.

Make sure that you are adequately hydrated, fully rested, and engage in some form of movement every day.

WEIGHT LOSS

Todays "Ketogenic Diet" is all the rage for cancer and advanced disease. But the diet can cause significant weight loss changes. Anyone with a low BMI cannot be on a diet this restrictive, as their weight may decrease. Any weight loss of 5 pounds or more in one week is significant. There are many side effects of chemotherapy and radiation that may make it hard to eat, such as nausea, taste changes, and mouth sores. Fast weight loss usually causes the loss of lean muscle mass, which is needed to maintain strength. It's best to increase the amount of protein eaten to stop losing lean muscle mass when dropping weight. Most people need to maintain their muscle mass because there is a poorer prognosis for patients who lose their lean body mass at a very rapid rate. Most men feel that weight loss is a bigger issue than weight gain. Men tend to feel weaker.

The following supplements will help:

→ Raw Liver extract or Methylated B's as directed on label; raw liver and B's increase the appetite.
→ Vitamin D; 5,000 to 10,000 i.u. daily.
→ Vitamin A with carotenoid complex with natural beta-carotene; 10,000 i.u. or as directed.
→ Vitamin C; 10,000 Grams daily, or as directed.
→ Vitamin E as directed.
→ Zinc; 100 mg daily; do not exceed dosage. Antiviral, improves taste and smell.

WEIGHT GAIN

Exercise

Keep as active as possible. Staying physically active is important for weight management regardless of whether weight loss or gain is desired because regular movement helps maintain lean muscle mass. Consider walking as a main exercise form, as lactic acid is a byproduct of sore muscles, and this causes cancer and advanced disease to grow.

Use supplements to rebuild your body

Our food is so adulterated with GMOs, hormones, antibiotics and processed substances that it is difficult, if not impossible, to get proper nutrition in the food that we eat. Eating whole foods to get the nutrients is the best option for food. But, because so much of our food is adulterated, we have to take supplements to rebuild our bodies. Vitamins or herbal supplements come in many forms; pills, shakes, or powders.

Essential oils

According to Higley, the best weight loss oils are Slique Essence(IA), EndoFlex (TA) (applied to throat and under big toes), Joy (TA), and Motivation (TA), Grapefruit, Orange and Lemon.

T: Apply as indicated or auricular emotion points.

A: Inhale directly, or diffuse.

Mobile tracking devices may help track diet components

Mobile tracking devices, apps downloaded on the smartphones, can be used to keep an online food journal to track the number of calories taken in, type and duration of exercise, and types of calories, such as the amounts of carbs, proteins and fats. Online mobile tracking devices make it easy to effect changes in your diet, which is the goal of tracking.

After treatment, be prepared for a change. No one gets out of long-term treatment unscathed. Both mental and physical changes linger after treatment. These changes may be weight loss or gain or some other complication. Mother knows best, she always said that eating a variety of good foods is best for health.

DYSPHAGIA OR TROUBLE SWALLOWING

Dysphagia is trouble swallowing when it is hard to get food or drink down the throat. Gagging, coughing, or choking is common, or a feeling that food is stuck, when trying to swallow. This problem is common with head and neck cancer and radiation to the breast or chest, or surgery involving the larynx. Trouble swallowing may be caused by radiation, surgery, or less commonly, chemotherapy.

Side Effects of Cancer or Advanced Disease Treatment

1. Fibrosis or scarring or stiffness in the throat, esophagus, or mouth.
2. Oral Mucositis is soreness, pain, or inflammation in the throat, esophagus, or mouth.
3. Structural changes, swelling or narrowing of the mouth, jaws, throat, or esophagus occur after radiation or surgery.
4. Dry mouth (Xerostomia) may occur from radiation therapy or chemotherapy, or from hormones.

For trouble swallowing:

- Eat soft, bland foods; moisten dry foods with sauces, gravies, broth, sauce, butter, or milk. Puddings, ice cream, soups, applesauce, and bananas and other soft smooth foods are easier to swallow.
- Mash or blend solid foods.
- Try thickening liquids. Add gelatin, tapioca, baby rice cereal, or commercial thickening products.
- Move your head back or forward while you are eating.
- Take a sip of water every few minutes to help you swallow and talk more easily. Carry a water bottle with you so you always have some handy.
- Use a straw to drink liquids and soft foods.
- Eat cold or room-temperature foods to reduce pain.
- Take small bites. Chew slowly and thoroughly.
- Eat small, frequent meals.
- Avoid foods that require a lot of chewing.
- Sit upright when eating or drinking.
- Choose foods high in calories and protein if you are **losing weight**. This includes eggs, casseroles, and nutritional shakes.
- Avoid dry, coarse, or hard foods.
- Drink meal replacement or nutritional supplement beverages.

Find the approach that works best as the severity and cause of swallowing problems affects the outcome. Multiple different therapies above may have to be tried to discover what works best. Try to eat a nutritious diet with enough calories, protein, vitamins, and minerals.

BOWEL AND BLADDER CONTROL

Bowel and bladder control issues are difficult physically and emotionally. The inability to adequately control and self-manage these is the number one reason that people are placed in nursing homes. Inability to control these often lead to social isolation, depression and self-loathing. Individuals often feel ashamed or fearful to go out in public. Medical doctors don't often discuss these problems. Bowel and bladder control loss can happen after any bladder, prostate, colon, rectal, ovarian, or other treatment. Constipation is most commonly caused by pain medication.

Ostomies are difficult to self-manage so there are services and support groups available to cope with these changes.

EndoFlex Oil applied over the kidneys as a hot compress may help.

- Radiation therapy to the pelvis (including reproductive organs, the bladder, colon and rectum) can irritate the bladder and urinary tract.
- Some types of chemotherapy and immunotherapy can also affect or damage cells in the bladder and kidneys.
- Surgery to remove the prostate (prostatectomy), bladder cancer surgery, and hysterectomy surgery, the tissue on the sides of the uterus, the cervix, and the top part of the vagina (radical hysterectomy) can also cause urinary problems. These types of surgery may also increase the risk of a urinary tract infection.

An irritation of the bladder lining can cause the following:

- pain or a burning feeling when you urinate
- blood in your urine (hematuria)
- trouble starting to urinate or urinary retention
- feeling that you need to urinate urgently or frequently
- leaking a little urine when you sneeze or cough
- bladder spasms, cramps, or discomfort in the pelvic area

Urinary tract infection (UTI):

- pain or a burning feeling when you urinate
- urine that is cloudy or red
- a fever of 100.5 °F (38 °C) or higher, chills, and fatigue
- pain in your back or abdomen
- difficulty urinating or not being able to urinate

To combat this, take Cranberry Pills as directed to change the pH of the bladder to alkaline. Lemon in 8oz of tap water makes alkaline water. Take 1 teaspoon of colidal silver every 8 hours.

A UTI can turn into a serious condition that needs immediate medical care or sepsis (an infection throughout the body) may occur. Antibiotics will be prescribed for bacterial infections by a medical doctor.

MENOPAUSE SYMPTOMS OR *"CHEMOPAUSE"*[29]

Menopause occurs naturally in women as hormones decline with age. It can also happen suddenly when reproductive organs are removed. Some cancer or advanced treatments can reduce the amount of hormones the woman creates by the ovaries, thus causing "chemopause." Sometimes, the ovaries stop working on their own. All this leads to menopause symptoms which is the permanent ending of a female's menstruation and fertility. Other health problems, such as cardiac disease, dryness and thinning of the vaginal tissues which can cause pain during sex. Osteoporosis may occur after menopause, along with bladder and urinary problems. Osteoporosis is found when the pH is acid as the blood pulls both magnesium and calcium out of the bones, teeth, and hair to buffer the blood to a pH of 7.35.

According to Higley, to balance female hormones, use Cypress, Lavender, Orange, Fennel, Sage, Roman Chamomile, Angelica or Basil essential oils.

Menopause symptoms are often treated by hormone therapy. A medical doctor uses chemical drugs containing estrogen and progesterone. A naturopath may use bioidentical hormones or natural supplements. Hormone therapy may not be a viable treatment, as it can raise the risk of cancer recurrence. Bioidentical hormones from plant sources may also increase disease risk. Sometimes menopause symptoms from hormone therapies, such as tamoxifen, can occur.

Menopause presents with many symptoms. Some things that can make menopause worse are smoking, osteoporosis, unhealthy weight, not drinking enough water (drink half your weight in ounces of water daily). It is important to exercise daily, both weight-bearing and muscle strengthening to prevent osteoporosis. Supplements that support healthy bone development and hormonal balance may help pH. These can help prevent bone loss.

Some supplements that may help are:

- Vitamin D3
- Calcium
- Magnesium
- Vitamin C
- Beta Glucans

Symptoms of Menopause:

1. Absent or Irregular periods; Periods become less regular, lighter and occasional with heavier bleeding.

2. Hot flashes feel like a hot oven door is open and the hot air hits you. According to Higley, to decrease hot flashes, use Peppermint, Clary Sage(estrogen), Bergarmot (estrogen), Fennel, or Dragon Time Essential Oils.

3. Vaginal Tissues become drier and thinner which cause infections in your vagina. Urinary tract problems or problems holding your urine also occur as decreasing hormones affect the bladder. According to Higley, try using Cypress mixed with V-6 oil over abdomen.

4. Hormonal decreases cause lower libido (sex drive) which means it is difficult to become sexually aroused. According to Higley, to increase libido, use Goldenrod, Lady Sclarol, or Ylang Ylang Oils. Maca can also be used at 500 mg per day.

5. Insomnia and fatigue, getting up early, or getting back to sleep after waking up in the middle of the night. Frequently the urge to urinate caused by the decrease in hormones awakens people during the night causing difficulty getting back to sleep, thereby causing tiredness during the day.

6. Hormonal declines cause memory problems and mood changes. They frequently occur at night, causing night sweats, sleep disruptions, and brain fog, which causes indecisiveness There may be a connection between changes in hormone level declines and depression, mood swings, and irritability, as emotions are affected. According to Higley, try Acceptance or forgiveness, brain power, Lavender, or Gathering.

7. Weight changes as the waist gets bigger with less muscle tone, increased fat, thinning and loss of elasticity in the skin.

Relieving menopause symptoms

a. Sleep on a ChiliPad (TN) in a cool room
c. Dress in layers that can be removed
d. Use cotton sheets and clothing
e. Drink something cold (water)
f. Try not to eat a lot of spicy foods.
g. Limit alcohol and caffeine intake
h. To decrease vaginal pain, use a lubricant, or Young Living Essential Oil Sensation. For vaginal inflammation use a vaginal moisturizer or, according to Higley, use Eucalyptus, Lavender, Melaleuca, or Yarrow.
i. For insomnia, according to Higley, use Lavender (best when used with Roman Chamomile, and Dill), RutaVaLa, Valerian, Bergamot, and Peace and Calming.

INTIMACY AND SEXUALITY

Sex after cancer can be complicated.[30] It is difficult in our society to talk about sex.

Sexual dysfunction after cancer treatment is a common issue for patients, says Dr. Karen Syrjala, co-director of Fred Hutchinson Cancer Research Center's Survivorship Program. "It depends on the diagnosis and type of treatment, but in prostate cancer we see sexual dysfunction in over 90 percent of men, and in women with breast cancer or bone marrow transplants, we see rates that are around 70 percent." In a 2010 Livestrong report, 43 percent of the 3,000-plus cancer patients surveyed had physical problems related to sexual functioning, and only 13 percent received help for them. You have to ask for help.

Sexual dysfunction is often caused by the changes experienced from surgery, chemotherapy, or radiation, or by the side effects of pain medicine. These problems cause depression, feelings of guilt about getting cancer, changes in body image after surgery, and stress between you and your partner.

Both men and women experience issues that come with receiving life-saving cancer and advanced disease treatment which can decrease your libido, make sex painful (or impossible), decrease ability to reach orgasm and even render your vaginas and penises numb. A nipple-sparing mastectomy eliminates sexual feeling with no nerves in the breast. Prostate cancer decreases a man's ability to achieve an erection. Cancer makes it difficult to have sex, as natural sexual lubrication is absent. The ability for response is diminished (or absent) with the physiological, emotional and/or psychological changes brought on by diagnosis and treatment. When death is imminent, it is hard to think about sex.

Chemotherapy and radiation damage the mucous membranes in your mouth, nose, eyes, ears, vagina, penis and anus. Radiation can cause skin burns, kill off the ovaries and sperm, and turn soft, sensitive tissue, thick and tough. Anti-hormone treatments, used with breast and prostate cancer patients, reduce blood flow, which can cause delicate tissues to atrophy.

After cancer and advanced disease treatment, sexuality and intimacy are affected and most doctors will not bring up sexual disfunction as it is often too uncomfortable. Patients that have been treated may live decades after treatment without sexual intimacy intact.

Diana's experience after treatment: I'd been married for 32 years when I was diagnosed with ovarian cancer. Suddenly, I was surgically post-menopausal, bald, had a misshaped breast, no libido and a painful vagina. While the doctor told me that my hair would fall out, no one mentioned that my eyebrows, pubic hair and even the leg and toe hair would fall out, as well. After surgery, I had drains bilaterally and was so thin I had no energy, down from140 to 100 pounds. My husband would hold me and kiss my bald head and I would just cringe. I felt very unattractive.

David, my husband, was my caregiver and I was his patient. He had trouble leaving that role as caregiver when my treatment was over. While treatment never ended for me, I learned and adapted to a "new way of life." For him, things were eternally different. No longer did he see me as his wife—I became a responsibility. I was no longer the sexual partner he once knew, as key parts of my sexual anatomy had been surgically removed. This had a profound impact on our quality of life as a couple. When we tried to renew our fractured relationship, I would get a new diagnosis of cancer somewhere else. The MD Anderson doctor that treated my stage-4 cancer never treated me as if I were going to survive; in fact, I was told that I might have as few as six months to live! My sexuality was not discussed—only the end of my life. Everything changed.

David and I have had to learn to live with sexual dysfunction. Somewhere along the way, with disappointment remembered, we realized that the old techniques do not work. We had to figure out how to fix it. I am now nine years out from diagnosis. To combat all this, I began taking NutriWest Core Level Ovary, and using Young Living Sensation for sexual intimacy.

According to Herron, "If there's pain or tenderness or lack of response, it becomes awkward and a "dead end" for couples. If that's the case for you and your partner, temporarily focus on intimacy rather than sex. Sometimes I'll tell patients to just leave the genitals out of it, and start with hand holding," she said. "There are other activities that might feel good – even just holding each other, rubbing each other, being physically sexual without having intercourse."

Sexual Options

1. Erection problems
    a. Penile Pump—implant in the penis with a pump bulb in the scrotum which will inflate the penis and then de-inflate it. It requires minor surgery.
    b. Goldenrod Oil apply to penis topically, SclarEssence taken in gelatin capsule 2-3 drops.

2. Infertility is the inability to have children. Some cancer treatments and advanced disease survivors permanently are unable to have children. Some possible solutions are egg harvesting or embryo freezing prior to treatment, or having a surrogate carry a child.

3. Fertility issues—a woman require to use birth control even if a period is not present. Women have been known to conceive while receiving cancer treatment.

4. Female arousal. There is a "little pink pill" called Addyi that has given some women good results. Essential Oils that are good options to increase desire are Lady Sclerol and Clary Sage, both applied topically.

5. Estrogen replacements—Are fine for some cancer patients; others could be harmful, but frequently, estradiol vaginal ring or vaginal suppositories or creams are acceptable. The vaginal area is like an estrogen sponge. If you use a topical estrogen product like an estring or an estrogen cream, it's incredibly unlikely you'll find that estrogen anywhere else in the body. (Natural Hormone Replacements are available such as NutriWest Core Level Ovary).

6. Kegal's exercises, will gain muscle and strengthen muscles in your genital area by doing these exercises. Practice by controlling your muscles to stop the flow of urine. You can do these exercises even when you are not urinating. Just tighten and relax the muscles as you sit, stand, or go about your day.

7. Decreased lubrication and blood flow to the genitalia causes atrophy, pain, loss of lubrication and lack of sensation. Special creams and ointments moisturize to reverse the effects of daily radiation.

8. Vibrators (most people have heard of these) or Dilators are useful for women who have had radiation or other damage to their vagina. They often come in a variety pack of sizes and, according to Heron, using them consistently "makes all the difference."

9. Also consider antidepressants, counseling, numbing creams or seeing a sex therapist. He or she may be able to help you talk openly about your problems, work through your concerns, and

come up with new ways to help you and your partner. Patients, partners and doctors don't always want to, or even know how to discuss sex, but communication is key.   Discuss this disfunction.[31]

CHAPTER 5: CANCER GROWS BACK FREQUENTLY AFTER CHEMOTHERAPY AS DAUGHTER CELLS AND STEM CELLS

"A cheerful heart is good medicine, but a crushed spirit dries up the bones."
- Proverbs 17:22

The reason conventional chemotherapy and conventional radiation have failed to change cancer survival rates is because cancer reproduces rapidly to create stem cells which divide asymmetrically, producing two daughter cells—one is a new stem cell and the second is progenitor cell, which can differentiate and proliferate, but cannot self-renew. Cancer stem cells are in all parts of your body like other stem cells.[32]

Cancer Stem Cells (CSC) become cancer daughter cells when these cancer cells multiply. They possess characteristics associated with normal stem cells. These may increase the growth, numbers, and strength of the cancer stem cells. While CSCs are only 1% to 3% of all cells in a tumor, they are the only cells with the ability to regenerate malignant cells and fuel the growth of the cancer.[33]

Daughter cells multiply to reproduce themselves and sustain cancer growth. Daughter cells are resistant to conventional chemotherapy and conventional radiation as a person is exposed to these. Conventional chemotherapy and conventional radiation damage the person's immune system and genetic systems as well as causing other side effects. These cells live in the bone marrow of long bones.

Anything taken by mouth is biochemical.

Some supplements strengthen the immune system to regrow the body's own killer cells to destroy cancer cells. We all have cancer cells, but they can be destroyed by a healthy immune system. Cancer cells produce Nagalase which is the substance that tells macrophages of the immune system to stay away. Genetic testing and other testing for any immune dysfunction must be corrected by effective support using specific nutrients, lifestyle changes, including regular daily sunshine, and highly restorative botanicals such as Beta-Glucans and mushroom complexes.

Genes that grow cancer or other advanced disease are changed by gene editing or changing those genes to resist cancer growth or advanced disease.

Daughter and stem cells can be defeated in the long bones by the following:

1. **Hyperthermia** is an immunological treatment where body tissue is exposed to high temperatures in order to damage and kill cancer cells.

An increase in body temperature is strongly correlated with a decrease in inflammation and survival from infection, cancer. This is illegal in the United States but not in Europe. Heat will kill daughter and stem cancer cells. The only legal heat machine sold in the US is the Photon Genius at a cost of $27,000.00. Many machines presently exist for hourly treatments; to find one near you, call The Skilling Institute, Arizona, for information on a machine owner near you. Dr. Ralf Kleef in Budapesh, Hungary has a variety of European hyperthermia machines.

2. **Coley's Toxins**

Dr. William Coley, the father of immunotherapy, developed a type of hyperthermia treatment for different types of bacteria to encourage the immune system to fight tumors. In 1891, Coley injected streptococcal organisms into a patient with inoperable cancer. Coley, a bone sarcoma surgeon, injected more than 1,000 cancer patients with bacteria or bacterial products. These products became known as Coley's Toxins. He and other doctors who used them reported excellent results, especially in bone and soft-tissue sarcomas. Coley's principles were correct in that some cancers are sensitive to an enhanced immune system. Coley's Toxins came under a great deal of criticism; many doctors did not believe his results.

3. **IV Vitamin C** – intravenous Vitamin C in large doses (50 to 150 Grams) will remove daughter and stem cells in the long bones.

DIET

Processed food is junk food. Most of us think of junk food as soft drinks, candy, snacks, fast food, and tv dinners. But in reality, junk food is almost any food that has been altered by man and packaged for resale. The best nutrition advice I've ever heard is this: **"If man made it, don't eat it." – Jack LaLane.**

According to Chris Wark, the nutritional value in the food that the food industry produces is decimated or destroyed. Processed food is loaded with artificial ingredients created in laboratories that we were never intended to ingest.

Chemical additives like artificial flavors, colors, and sweeteners make it look and taste good.

Chemical preservatives are added to make it last longer on the shelf. Then, synthetic vitamins and minerals are added to restore the nutritional value destroyed by all the processing.

Look at the ingredients on the labels of the food in your pantry.

If the label has ingredients you have never heard of, or cannot pronounce, beware. No processed food product can match the nutritional value of vitamins and minerals contained in raw organic fruits, vegetables, seeds, and nuts.

There's no way the FDA can test the long-term effects that all these artificial ingredients combined have on the human body over a lifetime, because everybody is different, and we are all eating different combinations of these artificial substances every day.

Unhealthful diet and lifestyle are proven causes of many diseases. Couple that with the fact that we live in a toxic world and we're constantly bombarded with invisible toxins that we can't see or avoid, and the problem is compounded. This is why it's increasingly important to limit the amount of toxins we ingest via the food we consume and the products we use.

The bottom line is that they are concerned with the bottom line. The commercial food industry exists to make money and they don't care about your health. The cheaper the ingredients, the more profit for the company. Unfortunately, the result is processed food with negative nutritional value loaded with sugar, salt, and toxic artificial colors, flavors and preservatives.

Simply put, cooking destroys enzymes, reduces the nutritional value of food, and raises its carcinogenic level. Whether you're in a lab or in the kitchen, subjecting any object to high heat causes a chemical reaction in that food which changes its structure. Cooking can convert nutrients from an organic to an inorganic state and render them useless nutritionally. Raw food is living food. Cooked food is dead. Raw food is perfectly designed to fuel a living body. The more raw food you can incorporate into your diet, the better.

Despite the millions of dollars spent by the food industry to convince us that "milk does a body good" and beef is "real food for real people," conventionally-produced meat and dairy are not healthful foods. The methods by which these foods are produced significantly degrade their nutritional value. Cows, chickens, and pigs are pumped full of steroids and antibiotics, live in cages covered in their own filth and are forced to eat corn-based feed instead of grass to fatten them up. This "conventional" meat is unusually high in fat and toxicity. Most of the fish consumed today is not caught in the wild. They are raised in chemical-filled pools at fish farms and fed an unnatural corn-based diet.

Most commercial dairy products are pasteurized and homogenized. These two processes radically transform milk into an unnatural form wholly unsuited for our bodies. Meat and dairy are acid-forming. The higher your internal acidity, the more susceptible you are to disease.

Meat and dairy are very rich foods with no fiber. The high protein can encourage disease cell growth, and they move through your digestive system very slowly, putrefying and releasing toxins back into your system. Cut them out of your diet completely while battling cancer or advanced disease.

Finally, grains are carbohydrates and carbohydrates are sugar.

A high-grain diet is a high-sugar diet. Sugar triggers an insulin release which converts excess sugars to be stored as fat and raises cholesterol, which can lead to weight gain, diabetes, cardiovascular disease. Elevated blood sugar increases tumor metastasis.

Wellness = nutrition + supplements + detoxing + excercise.

CHAPTER 6: ALKALINE WATER

"He said, "If you listen carefully to the Lord your God and do what is right in his eyes, if you pay attention to his commands and keep all his decrees, I will not bring on you any of the diseases I brought on the Egyptians, for I am the LORD, who heals you." - Exodus 15:26

Water is a key part of life and living. Your body is comprised of 70% water and it is critical that the water you drink when you have cancer or advanced disease be clean, pure and alkaline. It is difficult to determine water's purity, its source, its content, and its PH level. According to Robert Wright[34], "what we don't know or fail to realize is that most water is acidic, much of it is "dead" (no minerals), tap water is full of poisons (Chlorine and Fluoride), it struggles to hydrate our cells and contains oxidants rather than antioxidants...Increasing the alkalinity leads to decreasing the oxidants." To heal we must cleanse our bodies as much as possible, and this begins with clean, fresh, alkaline water.

Drink one half your weight in ounces of alkaline water daily (Ex: 100 pounds equal 50 ounces of water). Add additional alkaline water to the required amount above by adding the same number of ounces as any other drinks you have every day (Ex: If you drink 12 ounces coffee add 12 ounces of alkaline water in addition to the base number of ounces you need every day). To properly detox, you must have adequate water to flush your system of any metabolites from your liver and excreted them in your urine.

Stay Alkaline!

Alkaline water is water that has a high pH level (over 7.3) that makes it test alkaline versus any pH under 7.0 is acidic. Tap water is generally pH neutral or slightly acidic. Bottled water can be slightly alkaline or slightly acidic. It is believed that alkaline water slows aging, increases energy, regulates pH, and prevents disease. Alkaline water is less acidic than tap water and helps us to maintain an alkaline body.

Disease cells produce high acid levels in the body, so the Alkaline balance is disrupted by the acid produced by the disease cells.

A Kangen Water Machine costs about $4000.00, but it is responsible for healing many people of advanced disease. This is the best alkaline water machine on the market, according to Robert Wright.[35]

If you can't afford a Kangen Machine, use Bob's Red Mill Baking Soda stirred in a small glass of water twice a day. Be sure and test your alkalinity with PH Test Strips which you can buy at the pharmacy or order on line. The saliva should be about 6.8 or higher, and the urine at 7.0 or higher.

BAKING SODA

Baking soda's chemical name is sodium bicarbonate or sodium hydrogen carbonate. It is a white crystalline solid that appears as fine powder. The medical uses of baking soda all involve raising the pH of the body by neutralizing acid and treating acidosis (raise the pH level of the blood when it is close to 7.0).

Baking Soda (or sodium bicarbonate) decreases lactic acid. This same mechanism of increasing alkalinity and neutralizing acid and why baking soda is used in cancer treatment. Oral sodium bicarbonate is safe and can be readily used at home (make sure that the Baking Soda used has no Aluminum in it).

When mixed with a sweet substance such as honey, molasses, or maple syrup, the hungry cells open up to receive the Baking Soda and sweetener. Cancer prefers sugar so it does not have to break down food to grow.

Remember, without a hospitable body, the cells then die.

The Baking Soda Recipe to Alkalinize the Body

To make the baking soda natural cancer remedy at home, you need maple syrup, molasses or honey to go along with the baking soda. Take when hungry on an empty stomach.

Day 1: Mix 1 teaspoon of baking soda with 1 teaspoon of molasses in a cup of water. Take daily.

Day 3: Test the saliva with pH strips. The saliva pH should read 7.0 and the urine pH should read higher, at 7.3 to 7.5.

Day 5: Take the solution twice on Day 5 instead of once daily.

Day 6 – 10: Take 2 teaspoons each of baking soda and sweetener twice daily.

To Make Boiled Baking Soda Mixed With Maple Syrup:

Mix 90 teaspoons of maple syrup with 30 teaspoons of baking soda. The maple syrup must be boiled down to become thicker (the color of caramel). Then the baking syrup is added and stirred for 5 minutes until it is fully dissolved.

This preparation should provide about 10 days' worth of the baking soda remedy. 5 – 7 teaspoons per day is the recommended dose.

THE USE OF BAKING SODA IN ONCOLOGY

Even though most oncologists do not recommend sodium bicarbonate for their patients, they actually use it for the same purposes in chemotherapy. By combining this alkalinizing agent with chemotherapy drugs, it protects the organs of the body from being destroyed by the poisonous effects of those drugs. Essentially, sodium bicarbonate raises the pH around these vital organs and prevents the cancer from spreading there and chemotherapy drugs from causing even greater destruction.

Clinical Evidence for the Efficacy of Baking Soda in Cancer Therapy

The study results showed that baking soda, indeed, raised the pH and reduced spontaneous metastases in mice induced with breast cancer. The researchers also determined that sodium bicarbonate works by raising the pH outside cells and not within cells. This is an important finding because it suggests that sodium bicarbonate does not interfere with cellular metabolism even as it makes the microenvironment unconducive for tumor growth.

This is the reason both the pH of the saliva and wine are taken to determine the intracellular and extracellular fluid levels.

Other findings from this study show that baking soda:

1. Reduces the involvement of the lymph node on the transport of cancer cells
2. Does not lower the levels of circulating tumor cells (Cimetadine does)
3. Reduces the involvement of the liver and, therefore, the spread of tumor cells to other organs
4. Inhibits the colonization of other organs by circulating tumor cells
5. Inhibits the spread of prostate cancer but not melanoma[36] according

to researchers who injected sodium bicarbonate in other animal models for cancer

FASTING—FAST-TRACK YOUR METABOLISM

You've probably heard that going without food for a few hours puts your body into "starvation mode," where all weight loss will stop, and you'll begin to waste away. Interestingly, studies show the opposite effect—metabolism actually increases during short-term "fasting" periods, by up to 10 percent. Fasting allows cells and organs to "clean house," so to speak, of toxins.

Water Fasting is fasting by drinking water only.

Benefits of Water Fasting:

1. Weight loss—Ketosis is the state in which your body begins using energy from your internal fat stores instead of food. Water fasting helps your body reach ketosis more quickly than dieting. When you refrain from consuming calories, your body is forced to burn fat cells for energy.[37] This also reduces cancer stem cells. Ketones (produced when carbohydrates are reduced) are used as a primary energy source that helps the body to cleanse and detoxify.

2. Immune System Improves as reduced inflammatory cytokines decrease inflammation in the body.

3. Slows Aging as fasting has been found to reduce oxidative damage.

4. Stimulates Cellular Autophagy as the body breaks down old damaged cells and eats them.

5. Destroys and recycles damaged tissues as fasting can encourage your body's natural healing mechanisms.

6. Energy Conservation that reduces digestive inflammation as the need for energy for the digestive system, the immune system, tissue regeneration, physical movement (kinetics), to maintain mental focus, and to carry out many other activities. Digestion stimulates inflammation.

7. Helps healing as when healing from an illness, as much energy as possible is devoted toward the immune system and tissue

regeneration. This is why: when people are ill they naturally lose their appetite.

8. Improves Genetic Repair Mechanisms as it increases human growth hormone (HGH) which creates metabolic changes that burn fat and spare muscle. Fasting begins to focus on tissue repair (the body uses amino acids and enzymes to repair tissue collagen), which increases function of the muscles, tendons, ligaments, and bones.

9. Improves Insulin Sensitivity as fasting has been shown to reduce insulin secretion and improve cellular insulin sensitivity. Fasting lowers glucose and IGF1.

10. Drink High-Quality Water two or more quarts per day of fresh, clean, high-quality water.

Water Fasting Tips:

1. Make a schedule. If possible, take time off work. Decide on a length of time for your water-fasting cancer cleanse. Fasts can be done for any length of time up to about a month. You may consider a supervised water fast at a fasting clinic. They can do tests to monitor your health and help ease you back to solid foods.

2. Rest frequently, as fasting is a time for rest. The body will want to sleep more than usual. Listen to your body; you may need 12 hours or more of sleep each night, and naps during the day. Dr. Johanna Budwig of the Budwig Diet, thought rest was imperative to regaining health.

3. Difficulty: The first three days are going to be the worst, as the cells open up and dispel all the toxins they have stored over the years. Symptoms may include hunger, irritability, headaches, or disorientation. Fortunately, the body is resilient and should quickly adapt. The third or fourth day is better as the toxins are gone. Many people even report a feeling of euphoria at this point.

4. Break your fast slowly. Start by drinking only juices and detox waters, then broths, and gradually add in solid foods. Breaking the fast can be a multi-day process for longer fasts.

STRENGTHENING THE IMMUNE SYSTEM DIET

A diet of 80% fresh vegetables and juice, whole grains, seeds, nuts and a little fruit help put the body into an alkaline state. 20% can be from cooked food, including beans. Fresh vegetable juices provide live enzymes that are easily absorbed and get down to cellular levels within 15 minutes to nourish and enhance growth of healthy cells.

Eating with your hands as a guide to wellness

To eliminate calorie counting, use your hand as a guide for portion control.

The **palm** of your hand indicates how much protein you need at every meal. The **fist** of your hand indicates how much vegetables you need at a meal. A **hand full** indicates how much cooked carb-dense food you can eat. A **thumb** is the amount of fat usually eaten. Always remember to eat good fat such as that found in bananas, avocados, coconut oil, nuts, olive oil, avocado oil, almond oil, eggs, butter, and other Medium Chain Triglycerides (MCTs).

The size of **your** hand indicates the size of **your** portions.

Moderate Protein – Use your palm to measure

Proteins are complex organic acids that you must take in every day because you cannot absorb all amino acids in your food. Without amino acids, nothing else absorbs completely. Proteins provide energy for the body and are an important component of every cell. Nails are made of mostly protein.

Eat palm-sized or up to 6 ounces organic fat and protein foods three to four times a day.

Eat organic, free-range meats: Poultry, Beef, Lamb, Fish, Shellfish, Eggs

Cheese and Nuts, Use your thumb to measure

Thumb size: Cheeses such as cheddar, cottage, jack, mozzarella, goat, brie

Nuts: almonds are alkaline. Use caution with peanuts as they frequently have high levels of fungus, so only use organic peanuts and peanut butter. But all nuts are acceptable. Nuts are associated with improved outcomes when 2 ounces per day are eaten.

Protein drinks such as the Adkins and other available brands can be used; just make sure that there are not high levels of sugar and the drink is made with Stevia and not Aspartame or Splenda or any other chemical sweetener.

Avoid any sweetener with "mal" in the name, as this is also not good for people with cancer and advanced disease. Protein drinks help maintain nutrients and repair tissue.

Flaxseeds are critical Omega 3s that can help rebuild the body.

Acceptable Carbohydrates

½ cup or ½ fist, unprocessed brown rice per day at only one meal, preferably the noon meal is acceptable.

Flavorings

All spices and flavorings are to be used as desired. Spices are beneficial for rebuilding the body. Use garlic and onions as desired.

Use Celtic or Himalayan salt for mineral content and do not use table salt.

Take Iodine supplements.

Fruits

Lemons and limes are also to be used as desired. Make lemonade with Stevia.

One fresh orange a day is allowed. Strawberries, blueberries, blackberries, black raspberries, sour cherries, cranberries, pomegranates, and raspberries are allowed. Try them as a light dessert with whipped cream made with Stevia.
A small bowl of mixed berries such as strawberries, raspberries, blackberries, and blueberries with real whipped cream (no artificial anything) sweetened with Stevia is antioxidant-rich and flavorful.

Dark chocolate over 70% Cocoa in small amounts. Absolutely no milk chocolate.
Olives

Eat 4 black or green organic olives each day for the fat content.

Vegetables—as much as desired

Eat as many leafy green vegetables as you desire every day: spinach, broccoli, broccoli shoots, cauliflower, brussels sprouts, cabbage, celery, peppers (red, yellow, and green), kale, asparagus, green beans, eggplant, yellow squash, mustard greens, collard greens, turnip greens, okra, parsley, lettuce (except iceberg), carrots, and watercress. You can have green peas on occasion.

Liquids

Remember: Add pure ionized alkaline water, free of chlorine, which should equal half your weight in ounces of water, plus however, any ounces for other fluids you drink.

Plus white teas, peppermint teas, red teas (rooibos), black tea, herbal teas, fresh lemonade with stevia, V8, fruit juice you make yourself (preferably mixed with vegetables). Drink green tea. The ECGC in the green tea is wonderful for rehydrating the body. Let the green tea seep for 5-7 minutes.

It is critical that you own a Magic Bullet or other high-speed type blender that breaks down the cell walls of the vegetables and fruits so that you can prepare fresh green smoothies to get additional servings of fresh green vegetables that are easily digestible. Raw foods contain enzymes that dissipate when cooked. I frequently make a "liquid salad" by blending kale, celery, cucumber, carrots, broccoli, and any other vegetable, and drinking it with my lunch.

Coffee is hotly debated as a drink that is acceptable as it puts undue stress on the adrenal glands. When you make Organic coffee with 9.5 Alkaline water from a ionized water machine such as a Kangen, the coffee has a PH of 7 to 7.5. I feel that one to two cups of coffee made this way and consumed within 30 minutes of brewing will force the body to metabolize fatty acids to burn as energy which increases effectiveness of the diet. The coffee cannot sit longer than 30 minutes or it will become too acidic, and we want to maintain an Alkaline PH.

If you are still concerned about coffee, you can order Ganoderma Coffee or a similar brand. This is a premium coffee made from coffee beans and Ganoderma Lucidium mushrooms (Red Reishi). The mushrooms have antioxidant properties that improve health and strengthen the immune system. Mushrooms should be a part of every recovery patients' protocol. Mushrooms are known to decrease stress, toxins, infections, and improve respiration and circulation while improving the immune system.

I have tried the Ganocafe Classic and was not thrilled to be ordering instant coffee, but it has proven handy when traveling. It was almost as good as the organic coffee that I make at home. Remember that Ganocafe is an alkaline product. You can order it at www.GanoExcel.us

Diana's Coffee[38] to decrease Inflammation

Coffee made with alkaline water to increase pH
2 or 3 Tablespoons Coconut Oil
Coconut Creamer to taste
Sprinkle Cinnamon, Cayenne Pepper, Turmeric, and Cocoa powder in coffee. Stir and drink.

Oils

Fat is metabolized as fat or ketones. The optimal fats are the Medium Chain Triglycerides (MCT) which are hemp oil, coconut oil, coconut butter, avocados, macadamia nuts, butter, eggs and other saturated fats. These MCTs are easier to convert to ketones by the body than polyunsaturated fats.

Olive oil as desired, 4-6 tablespoons butter (no margarine), coconut oil or coconut cream, (you can eat coconut oil by the spoonful if you desire), avocado, organic nut butters such as almond, or walnut, ground flaxseed (use within 15 minutes of grinding, as flax seeds loose effectiveness and become rancid), organic raw or dry-roasted seeds such as pumpkin seeds, sesame seeds (unhulled), squash seeds, sunflower seeds.

Black Seed Oil from Turmeric

Black Seed Oil or *N. sativa* is a flowering plant that lives in India and the Mediterranean and Middle East regions with medicinal uses for diabetes, migraines, cancer, and advanced disease. The plant's seeds, also called black cumin, contain a potent compound called thymoquinone that has anti-inflammatory and antioxidant properties. The oil extracted from black cumin seeds has been studied extensively, and findings show that it both prevents and treats disease.[39]

The Budwig Diet with Cellect or Trican Powder = BALANCED FATS

Dr Johanna Budwig was nominated 6 times as a Nobel Prize winner and a world leader of her time in essential fatty acids and fat absorption. She developed The Budwig Diet, discovering that essential fatty acids combine with sulphur-rich proteins to increase oxygenation in the body which limits the growth (metastasis) of cancer cells. Dr. Budwig treated cancer patients in the last hours of life and is reported to have a cure rate of over 90% of terminally ill patients. The Budwig Diet is one of the best known, oldest, and most established alternative treatments for cancer with **NO side effects.**

While it can be classified as an oxygen treatment plan, its actual mechanism is to reverse mitochondrial respiratory suffocation and force oxygen into the cancer cells, which not only kills them, but does no harm to the normal cells. "The theory," says Budwig, "is the use of oxygen in the organism can be stimulated by protein compounds of sulphuric content, which make oils [Omega-3] water-soluble."

In short, this diet stops the spread of cancer and kills cancer cells. When you combine the Ketogenic Diet and the Budwig Diet, you have a strong mechanism for eliminating cancer and advanced disease.

Do not use any other oil except flaxseed oil. Fish oil has too many impurities. Coconut oil does not have the exact same mechanism. This diet needs to be measured precisely and taken for five years.

The Budwig mixture should be taken once or twice a day for five years. It should be stirred with a wooden or plastic spoon. Wood is ideal, and metal should never be used.

- 1 Tablespoon Flaxseed—ground in the Magic Bullet then poured into a bowl
- 2 Tablespoons Flaxseed Oil—Barleans is my favorite brand
- 4 Tablespoons Nancy's Low-Fat Organic Cottage Cheese

Mix the cottage cheese and flaxseed oil with a wood or plastic spoon in the magic bullet. You can thin it down with a little flax milk, coconut milk, or almond milk (but no other milk). Turn the bullet on and blend until the flaxseed oil and cottage cheese are completely blended together. The consistency should be like whipped cream, with no flaxseed oil floating on the sides of the bullet. Pour over ground flaxseeds in the bowl. You can add cinnamon, Stevia, berries, walnuts, almonds, macadamia nuts, garlic, cayenne, red pepper, or champagne.

Wait 5 minutes for the chemical reaction to complete; then eat within 15 minutes.

Use Nayonaise or Vegannaise as a substitute for Mayonnaise

No commercial salad dressings or toppings.

No commercial mayonnaise (bastardized, radioactive, genetically engineered, corn, canola and soy oils)

No butter, and especially no margarine or other artificial butters (Butter is normally extremely beneficial, but it will interfere with the Budwig Protocol). Substitute coconut oil.

Avoid the following fats:

Partially hydrogenated fats and oils, Trans Fats, Margarine, Lard, Corn Oil, Cottonseed Oil, Sunflower Oil, Palm Oil.

Avoid pure animal fats, such as lard, fatback, dripping, bacon and pork, etc. Fats are a myth perpetuated on the American people. Our healthy cells require Omega 3's to maintain their ability to carry on healthy cellular processes. We have been told that fats are bad for everyone, but for a person to heal, he must have a diet full of healthful fats.

As every cell in the body has 2 walls made only of fat.

Fats are critical for the Ketogenic Diet as the fats turn more easily into ketones.

Sweeteners

Sweeteners go through the water treatment system, so you get these even when you don't eat them. Be aware.

Stevia is the only sweetener that is safe at this time. Do not use Aspartame—the data is overwhelming that this is an horrific poison, as just look it up on the Internet. Splenda is known to cause an allergic reaction in up to 70% of women and is unhealthful.

Sugar will feed cancer and advanced disease and will shut down the immune system for at least 30 minutes. Sugar is not permitted on the Ketogenic Diet and will throw you out of ketosis.

Avoid all artificial sweeteners (including high-fructose corn syrup).

Snack

Try to combine fiber and protein to satisfy your hunger.

1. Celery with almond or walnut butter, or cheese
2. Cherry Tomatoes with mozzarella cheese
3. Veggies with hummus
4. Deviled eggs made with Veganaise instead of Mayonnaise
5. Guacamole-stuffed cherry tomatoes

Broth

Bone Broth is very healthful and healing. Always save your Organic bones and place in a slow cooker covered in water and simmer up to 2 days. This is very good to cook rice in or to drink to satisfy hunger.

Organic broth can be purchased from the grocery store.

Apple Cider Vinegar

You must consume 2 tablespoons Apple Cider Vinegar every day as ACV Tea (a cup of water with 2 tablespoons apple cider vinegar and Stevia to sweeten). Or use apple cider vinegar as a salad dressing or on vegetables.

Additional Tips

1. Eat an entirely chemical-free diet, organic.
2. Avoid all processed foods.
3. Attempt to wean off of all pharmaceuticals with the help of a medical doctor.
4. Avoid all soft drinks.
5. Avoid tap water and bottled water, and use products free of fluoride.
6. Eat all foods freshly prepared. No reheating and no leftovers.
7. Make and inventory all chemicals that touch your skin, and stop using anything that is not organic and pure. Anything that touches your skin will be absorbed in 28 seconds!

Protein Powder

A really delicious breakfast is ½ cup Oatmeal, 2 scoops chocolate protein powder, and a spoon of organic peanut butter. This tastes like a Reese's Peanut Butter Cup.

Increase Enzymes

To obtain live enzymes for building healthy cells, try drinking fresh vegetable juice (most vegetables, including bean sprouts) and eat some raw vegetables 2 or 3 times a day. Enzymes are destroyed at temperatures of 104 degrees F (40 degrees C), so do not cook these.

Cancer cell walls have a tough protein covering. By refraining from or eating less meat it frees more enzymes to attack the protein walls of cancer cells and allows the body's killer cells to destroy the cancer cells.

Include: Supplements that will strengthen the immune system, such as Beta glycans and vitamin C.

Avoid: Sugar substitutes like NutraSweet, Equal, and Spoonful made with Aspartame, which are all harmful and weaken the immune system.

Instead: A better natural substitute would be coconut sugar, manuka honey or molasses, but only in very small amounts.

Avoid: Table salt, which has an additive for bleaching.

Instead: Better alternative is Bragg's amino acid or Celtic or Himalayan salt.

Avoid: Milk causes the body to produce mucus in the gastro-intestinal tract. Dairy products contain high levels of growth hormones and antibiotics and have been fed a diet of corn which is a Genetically Modified Organism (GMO), which kills all friendly bacteria in the gut. Cancer and advanced disease feed on mucus.

Instead: Substitute unsweetened coconut, Flax, or almond milk so no mucus is produced. Substitute unsweetened soy milk if you have Prostate cancer or can be sure that it is unadulterated, so no mucus is produced.

Avoid: Eating an acidic, meat-based diet (disease cells thrive in an acid environment). Meat also contains livestock antibiotics, growth hormones and parasites, which are all harmful, especially to sick people. Meat protein is difficult to digest and requires a lot of digestive enzymes. Undigested meat remaining in the intestines becomes putrefied and leads to more toxic waste buildup.

Instead: Eat fish, and a little white meat, like chicken.

To heal it is best to avoid dairy and gluten unless you have been allergy-tested and know that you have no sensitivities. It is possible to damage the cell lining of the small and large intestine which focuses the immune system on the gut instead of on rebuilding the body.

Most people have to supplement amino acids as they cannot get them in the adulterated food. Therefore, eat organic as much as possible to avoid chemicals that are added to meat.

CALORIE RESTRICTION AND DIETARY LIMITS

Overall calorie restriction is eating less of everything which is critical for cancer prevention and advanced disease.

Step 1—Set Carbohydrate limit at 12-25 Carbs daily

Step 2—Set Protein limit at 1.0 Protein/kg of lean body mass daily (3 servings a week of red meat).

No alcohol for three weeks, then one glass of red wine. White wine has NO therapeutic effect. It is the same as drinking vodka and Kool aid.

A normal day of eating should look like this:
Weight should not be gained or lost eating three meals with two snacks.

Breakfast: Budwig diet first thing in the morning topping with spices and fruit to balance your fats for the day.

Snack: A green drink after two hours.

Lunch: A raw vegetable salad topped with egg or some type of protein, or cooked homemade soup for lunch, no carbs. Or more Green drink, as this is a blended salad.

Snack: A green drink after two hours

Supper: One meat, and two vegetables. No fried food.

INTERMITTENT FASTING

The Standard American Diet (SAD Diet) is high in carbohydrates and the wrong kinds of fat so most people burn carbohydrates for fuel. To recover your health, shift your body from burning carbohydrates to burning fats (ketones) and restrict all eating to a 6-8-hour window, have no food after supper, and allow 3 hours between your last bite and bed. This upregulates the enzymes designed to burn fat and downregulates glucose.

Intermittent fasting is a terrific regulator of the immune system as it controls the levels of inflammatory cytokines that are released in the body. Two major cytokines are Interleukin-6 (IL-6) and Tumor Necrosis Factor Alpha (TNF-alpha)promotes potent inflammatory responses in the body. Fasting reduces the release of these inflammatory mediators and decreases allergies.

The normal person is infested with viruses, bacteria, fungi, and/or parasites. Intermittent fasting stimulates autophagy processes, which decrease viral, bacterial, and fungal infections and decrease the growth of intracellular parasites. Intermittent fasting's catabolic process helps the body rid itself of intracellular pathogens as well as halting abnormal cell development. It is also important in protecting the brain and tissue cells from abnormal growth, toxicity, and chronic inflammation.

Intermittent fasting is important, as it requires less energy to repair a cell than to divide and create new ones.

HOW TO DO INTERMITTENT FASTING

Intermittent fasting is going from 12 to 36 hours without food, not eating until lunch, then eating supper within 6-8 hours while avoiding eating anything 3 hours before bed.

Intermittent fasting starves cancer cells and leaves them vulnerable to free radical damage and ultimate destruction so they can die.

The time between your last meal of one day and the first meal of the next day can be called the "fasting window." Be sure to drink 8 to 16 ounces of water at a minimum when you first wake up to help reduce morning hunger, prolong the fast, and improve the cleansing process. You can drink Diana's Bullet Proof Coffee, and ACV Tea as a kidney flush.

GREEN JUICE FAST

Green Juice Fasts are green drinks without fruit in them other than lemons or limes, which contain few carbohydrates. Add an avocado to the green juice, as it allows emulsification and prevents juice separation. For example, add avocado while making a green juice with green lettuce, asparagus, lemon, celery, cucumber, kale, parsley, and ginger root to get nutrients into the body while also maintaining the benefits of the fast.

Diana's Green Drink (The Beast Slayer)

Start with 3 cups alkaline water and add 3 cups greens; blend until liquified. Then add all other vegetables, including an avocado or MTC oil. Add ½ cup fresh cranberries, ½ cup blueberries, and a banana, apple, or orange, if desired. Open spice cabinet and add ½ teaspoon Cinnamon, ½ teaspoon Cayenne, 1 teaspoon Turmeric and ½ teaspoon Celtic salt. These spices decrease inflammation and provide minerals.

CHAPTER 7: SUPPLEMENTS

My son, pay attention to what I say; turn my words. Do not let them out of your sight, keep them within your heart; for they are life to those who find them and health to one's whole body." - Proverbs 4:20-22

VITAMINS AND SUPPLEMENTS

A nutrient is referred to as a "vitamin" when it's essential for health, and our bodies cannot manufacture adequate quantities of it. We have to get vitamins through the diet or by taking a supplement. A vitamin needs to be present in its active form to perform its many jobs. Every vitamin is responsible for crucial roles in supporting health and wellness, and vitamins are often interdependent. Our bodies require 13 vitamins, eight of which make up the B-group (or B-complex) vitamins.

Make your body inhospitable to cancer and advanced disease by including additional vitamins and supplement balancers that are necessary.

To make your body inhospitable to cancer to cancer and advanced disease:

- → Balance vitamin D. Have that level drawn by your Medical Doctor each time lab is done. A physician from Germany feels that it is difficult for cancer to grow when vitamin D is 100.
- → Take vitamin D3 5000IU every day (get into an anticancer range of 86 or above. My experience is your body will stop supporting cancer at 86 or higher, so get your lab checked frequently)
- → The studies have shown increased survival in non-stem cell cancer treatment.
- → Amino Acids must be taken every day, as you cannot get the proper amino acids through the meat you eat. There is literature that claims that meat must be limited to starve out cancer, but to heal and absorb all vitamins and supplements, amino acids must be present with vitamin D.

Other Cancer and Advanced Disease Fighting Supplements that you need:

Grape Seed Extracts (Resveratrol and Procyanidins) have high concentrations of antioxidants, protecting the body against damage.

1. **Resveratrol**– Studies show this compound reduces the chances of harmful inflammation and free radical damage. It was also documented as slowing and even halting the development of tumors, especially those related to hormone imbalance (prostate or breast cancer).

2. **Procyanidins** – Like resveratrol, these antioxidants modulate inflammation and free radical damage. This includes the slowing down and reducing the chances of cancers and tumors.[40]

→ Take 500mg at Night.

Essiacs Tea either pills (I used the pills) or the tea. It is an herbal remedy that originated from a Canadian nurse, Marie Caisse, who used this blend for cancer. There are four herbs, which must be organic, that are typically used to make essiac tea: burdock root, sheep sorrel, slippery elm and Indian rhubarb root.

→ Take Morning and Night.

DIM Estro PM supports healthy estrogen metabolism in men and women. DIM is an advanced metabolite of Indole-3-Carbinol, the indole found in cruciferous vegetables.

→ Take as directed.

Alpha Lipoic Acid (ALA) can prevent certain kinds of cell damage and it restores vitamin E and C levels. It converts blood sugar (glucose) into energy using oxygen, a process referred to as aerobic metabolism. ALA is an antioxidant, meaning that it can neutralize harmful compounds called free radicals that damage cells at the genetic level.

→ Take 600mg Morning and Night.

Fractionated or Modified Citrus Pectin reduces tumor growth. According to Dr. Isaac Eliaz, Modified Citrus Pectin decreases the positively-charged ions (diseased) in the body and binds them, causing them to be flushed out of the body.

→ 2 scoops or pills a day on an empty stomach.

Beta Glucans act as immunomodulator agents; they cascade events to regulate the immune system which makes it more efficient.

→ Take as directed

B Vitamins

B vitamins are a class of water-soluble vitamins that play an important role in cell metabolism. There are 8 essential B vitamins, meaning that you cannot make these, but must get these from food or supplements. Note: These are important for healing.

→ Take as directed

List of Essential B vitamins[41]

B Number	Name	Discription
Vitamin B1	Thiamine	A coenzyme in the catabolism of sugars and amino acids.
Vitamin B2	Riboflavin	A precursor of cofactors called FAD and FMN which are needed for flavoprotein enzyme reactions, including activation of other vitamins.
B3	Niacin (nicotinic acid), Nicotinamide, nicotinamide Riboside	A precursor of coenzymes called NAD and NADP which are needed in many metabolic processes.
B5	Pantothenic acid	A precursor of coenzyme A needed to metabolize many molecules.
B6	Pyridoxine, pyridoxal, Pyridoxamine	A coenzyme in many enzymatic reactions in metabolism.
B7	Biotin	A coenzyme for carboxylase enzymes, needed for synthesis of fatty acids and in gluconeogenesis.
B9	Folate	A precursor needed to make, repair, and methylate DNA; a cofactor in various reactions; especially important in aiding rapid cell division and growth, such as in infancy and pregnancy.

B Number	Name	Discription
B12	Various Cobalamins; commonly Cyanocobalamin or Methylcobalamin in vitamin supplements	A coenzyme involved in the metabolism of every cell of the human body, especially affecting DNA synthesis and regulation, but also fatty acid metabolism and amino acid metabolism.

Vitamin	Name	Deficiency Effects
B1	Thiamine	Deficiency causes beriberi. Symptoms of this disease of the nervous system include weight loss, emotional disturbances, Wernicke encephalopathy (impaired sensory perception), weakness and pain in the limbs, periods of irregular heartbeat, and edema (swelling of bodily tissues). Heart failure and death may occur in advanced cases. Chronic thiamin deficiency can also cause alcoholic Korsakoff syndrome, an irreversible dementia.
B2	Riboflavin	Deficiency causes ariboflavinosis. Symptoms may include cheilosis (cracks in the lips), high sensitivity to sunlight, angular cheilitis, glossitis (inflammation of the tongue), seborrheic dermatitis or pseudo-syphilis (particularly affecting the scrotum or labia majora and the mouth), pharyngitis (sore throat), hyperemia, and edema of the pharyngeal and oral mucosa.
B3	Niacin	Deficiency, along with a deficiency of tryptophan causes pellagra. Symptoms include aggression, dermatitis, insomnia, weakness, mental confusion, and diarrhea. In advanced cases, pellagra may lead to dementia and death (dermatitis, diarrhea, dementia, and death).

Vitamin	Name	Deficiency Effects
B5	Pantothenic acid	Deficiency can result in acne and paresthesia, although it is uncommon.
B6	Pyridoxine, Pyridoxal, Pyridoxamine	Deficiency causes seborrhoeic dermatitis-like eruptions, pink eye and neurological symptoms (e.g. epilepsy)
B7	Biotin	Deficiency does not typically cause symptoms in adults but may lead to impaired growth and neurological disorders in infants. Multiple carboxylase deficiency, an inborn error of metabolism, can lead to biotin deficiency even when dietary biotin intake is normal.
B9	Folic acid	Deficiency results in a macrocytic anemia, and elevated levels of homocysteine. Deficiency in pregnant women can lead to birth defects.
B12	Cyanacobalamin	Deficiency results in a macrocytic anemia, elevated methylmalonic acid and homocysteine, peripheral neuropathy, memory loss and other cognitive deficits. It is most likely to occur among the elderly, as absorption through the gut declines with age; the autoimmune disease, pernicious anemia, is another common cause. It can also cause symptoms of mania and psychosis. In extreme cases, paralysis can result.

METHYLATED B VITAMINS

This is Super Important!

Methylated B vitamins—methylation has a significant positive impact on many biochemical reactions in the body that regulate the activity of the cardiovascular, neurological, reproductive, and detoxification systems, including those relating to DNA production, neurotransmitter production, detoxification, histamine metabolism, estrogen metabolism, eye health, fat metabolism, cellular energy, and liver health.

Determine if you have the MTHFR genes—have your genes tested.
A Methylated B, if you have positive gene for MTHFR: as directed.

Curcumin (Turmeric) has 48 anti-cancer effects. It has the best effects on breast cancer, bowel cancer, stomach cancer and skin cancer cells.

→ Take up to 10 grams per day - ten 1,000 mg tablets

Epigallocatechin gallate (ECGC)[42] studies support an association between ECGC consumption and a reduced cancer risk. These are used in combination with other supplements to increase the cancer over coming properties.

→ Take each as directed.

Heart:

Coenzyme Q10 (CoQ10) may help the immune system and is used as the primary treatment to increase the chances of a cure. CoQ10 may help slow tumor growth by immune augmentation, suppression of vascular endothelial growth factor (that facilitates tumor angiogenesis), and reduction of inflammatory markers that may facilitate cancer cell propagation. CoQ10 decreases treatment side effects.

Melanoma and breast cancer are two types of malignancies for which CoQ10 has demonstrated substantial clinical benefit. A recent melanoma study compared the effects of administering alpha interferon with or without daily CoQ10 (400 mg). There was an astounding 10-fold lower risk of metastasis in the CoQ10-supplemented group! This effect was even more pronounced for those with more advanced melanoma, where CoQ10-supplemented patients were 13 times less likely to develop metastasis.[43]

→ Take one at night

OMEGA 3 FATTY ACIDS

1. **Alpha-linolenic acid (ALA)**, ALA, derived from plants, is found in walnuts and other nuts, flaxseed, and other edible seeds, and in oils (e.g., canola, soy, hemp). Omega 3.
2. **Eicosapentaenoic acid (EPA)** Omega 3.
3. **Docosahexaenoic acid (DHA)**, a primary structural component of the human brain, cerebral cortex, skin, and retina.
   EPA and DHA are marine-based, and are sourced from salmon, tuna, trout, and other fatty fish, as well as phytoplankton and algae.[44]

→ One capsule, AM and PM

Vitamin E—(MUTLTI TOPHERICOLS) causes apoptosis or programmed cell death.

→ 800mg each morning

Essential Nutrients (your body doesn't make it):

Selenium

Selenium is an essential mineral that is a component of an antioxidant enzyme, glutathione reductase, and is part of tissue respiration.[45] It is also an important part of the immune system. The three forms of selenium most important in cancer prevention are ***sodium selenite, L-selenomethionine*** and ***selenium-methyl L-selenocysteine***, they complement one another by affecting your body's expression of important proteins involved in cancer prevention and suppression.[46]

→ Selenium 400 mg in Morning must be taken opposite of Zinc.

*Detailed studies now reveal the following **12** distinct mechanisms by which selenium prevents potentially cancerous cells from attaining full-blown tumor status:*

1. *Regulation of lipoxygenases, enzymes that produce inflammatory molecules that promote cancer growth;*
2. *Direct reduction of oxidative stress that causes free radical damage;*
3. *Protection of the antioxidant-recycling seleno-proteins;*
4. *Detoxification of cancer-inducing metals;*
5. *Induction of protective "phase II" liver enzymes that neutralize organic carcinogenic toxins;*
6. *Inhibition of DNA alterations, precursors to initiation of cancerous changes;*
7. *Inactivation of molecular transcription factors required by cancer cells to support their growth and development;*
8. *Shutting down of the essential cell replication cycle needed by cancer cells to produce their explosive growth;*
9. *Induction of apoptosis, the programmed cell death, a natural feature of all normal body cells that is missing in cancerous cells, allowing them to continue to reproduce indefinitely;*
10. *Enhanced immune system activity to detect and destroy incipient cancer cells;*
11. *Downregulation of sex hormone receptors used by certain cancers to sustain their growth;*
12. *Limiting effects on tumor invasion and metastasis.*

Zinc

Zinc improves immune functions while it acts as an antioxidant and anti-inflammatory agent. Oxidative stress and chronic inflammation have been implicated in many cancers. (In patients with head and neck cancer, nearly 65% were zinc-deficient based on their cellular zinc concentrations). Natural killer (NK) cell activity and IL-2 generation were also affected adversely. Zinc supplementation has beneficial effects on cancer by decreasing angiogenesis and induction of inflammatory cytokines while increasing apoptosis in cancer cells.[47]

Zinc decreases mucous production, especially during chemotherapy (cancer grows on mucous).

Zinc decreases dysgeria which are urinary tract infections.

→ 50 mg at night opposite of Selenium.

Improves digestion and support healthy immune system function:

Digestive Enzymes provide maximum absorption to break down the food we eat. We need assistance in breaking down protein, fats, and carbohydrates, as the water we drink has fluoride which depletes these enzymes.

→ Take as directed.

Magnesium

Magnesium studies show magnesium deficiency as a risk factor for some types of cancers and can hinder chemotherapy treatment.[48] Higher intakes of magnesium is correlated with lower risk of colorectal cancer (probably in part due to its efficiency in moving stool through the colon).[49]

Magnesium regulates nephrotoxicity during chemotherapy.

→ 1,500 mg at Night—if diarrhea begins, back down the magnesium.

Probiotics

Probiotics are highly beneficial live bacteria, viruses, and yeasts. This is an environment in which our healthy and pathogenic viruses and bacteria live, in what's called a symbiosis or a state of health and regulation. The microbiome is known to start in the gut, but our entire body is a microbiome.

After effects of cancer and advanced disease include:

1) Suppression of the growth of microbiota implicated in the production of mutagens and carcinogens
2) Alteration in carcinogen metabolism
3) Protection of DNA from oxidative damage
4) Regulation of immune system. Studies have shown that probiotics guard against the invasion of cancer cells, and reduces the likelihood of metastasis and other disease after effects.[50]

Probiotics can increase or decrease diarrhea, increase gas and bloating, and produce headaches and allergies. If you have proper detoxing the symptoms should be less extensive.

Fermented vegetables, yogurt, kombucha, kefir and **sauerkraut** are natural probiotics.

Chicory is the best natural probiotic. Take as directed.

Melatonin

Melatonin's Impressive Role in Fighting Cancer

Peer-reviewed and published research has shown that melatonin offers particularly robust protection against reproductive cancers.

Cells throughout your body, including cancer cells, have melatonin receptors.

Melatonin production peaks during the night which causes cell division to slow. When this hormone attaches to a breast cancer cell, it has been found to counteract estrogen's tendency to stimulate cell growth.

Melatonin has a calming effect on several reproductive hormones, which may explain why it seems to protect against sex hormone-driven cancers, including ovarian, endometrial, breast, prostate and testicular cancers.
While causing cancer cells to self-destruct, melatonin also boosts your production of immune-optimizing substances such as interleukin-2, which helps identify and attack the mutated cells that lead to malignant cancer.

According to Dr. Mercola, Melatonin's immediate precursor is the neurotransmitter, serotonin, which is a major player in regulating and giving a lift to your mood. Melatonin, like serotonin, plays an important role in your physical and mental health. Studies have shown that insufficient melatonin production can set you up for:

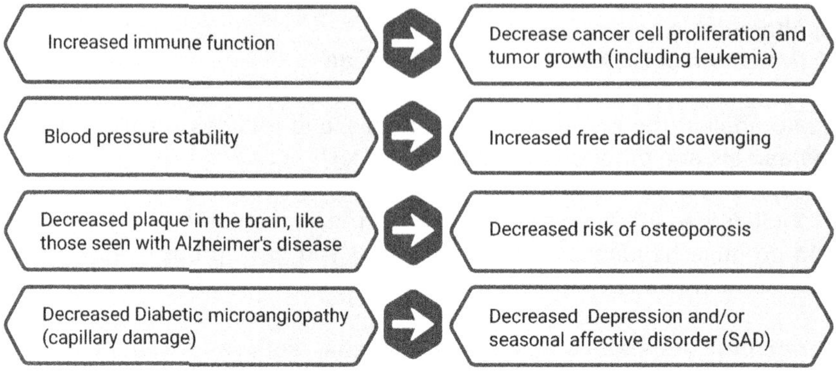

Neem

Immune Neem's beneficial properties include easy availability, low cost and safety to humans, tumor selectivity, and therapeutic safety. Its use in combination with other anticancer drugs is implicated in cancer therapy. Neem extracts deliver their anticancer efficacy by suppression of angiogenesis, cell migration and proliferation, and NF-κB signaling. The neem extracts enhance cell death, immunity against tumors, and cellular metabolism including modulation of redox potentials.[51]

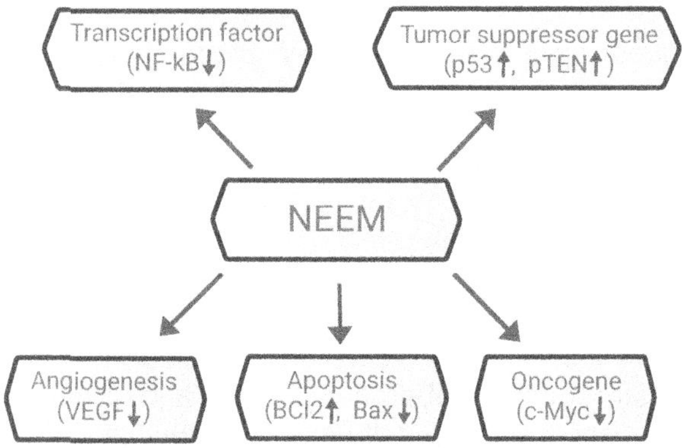

→ Take as directed or 1 capsule AM and PM

Anticoagulant and anticancer:

1) Baby Aspirin studies show a 23% decrease in Ovarian Cancer.
→ Take 83mg Baby Aspirin, every other day
2) Cinnamon and Alpha Lipoic Acid (ALA) stabilize energy in the absence of glucose. Use cinnamon liberally in drinks and on food. You can also take cinnamon capsules.

Other things that may be useful:

◆ **Quercetin** is a unique antioxidant that has been shown to have a profound effect on reducing oxidative stress and preventing and reversing cancer cell development. Quercetin reduces oxidative stress and inflammation, and protects the body from the development of chronic disease and cancer.

- About 400-1,200 mg/day

◆ **Sunshine** for vitamin D and enhanced well-being.

◆ **Cod Liver Oil** for constipation, rickets, and vitamin supplementation.

◆ **Wheat Grass and Barley Life** The green is from chlorophyll and helps to support the immune system with multiple nutrients such as vitamins, minerals, amino acids, antioxidants and enzymes. It is an Alkaline producing supplement that blocks free radical damage in essential fats such as omega-3 fatty acids, according to the Journal of Agricultural and Food Chemistry in 2012.

◆ **Iodine** is an essential element. It is part of thyroid function. Its role as an anticarcinogenic agent is just beginning to be widely appreciated. Iodine prevents cancers through antioxidant, anti-inflammatory, pro-differentiating, and pro-apoptotic effects. There is little risk to adding whole sea vegetables to the diet.

◆ **Chlorella** is a superfood. It is a single-celled stasis. This fresh water algae is rich in vitamins, minerals, amino acids, enzymes, and polysaccharides.

Research shows that chlorella:

1. *Delivers ten times the beta carotene of carrots and is a particularly high source of vitamin B-12*
2. *Offers 17 times the nucleic concentration of sardines, which is good for anti-aging and rejuvenation*
3. *Contains more chlorophyll per gram than any other plant, which increases oxygenation and helps provide the body magnesium*
4. *Includes polysaccharides which are shown to be essential in boosting the immune system and the ability for cells to communicate (in particular the presence of any rogue cells)*
5. *Has a fibrous wall, which helps chelate toxins in the blood stream and gut to move them out of the body*
6. *Can improve cellular glutathione levels and detoxify the cells of free-radicals*[52]

◆ **Colloidal silver** has been used as an antimicrobial and disinfectant agent for hundreds of years. Colloidal silver might be a potential alternative agent for human breast cancer therapy.[53]

◆ **Bentonite Clay** is a powerful antibacterial agent. Being highly charged with negative ions, it will naturally bond with substances that have a high positive charge, such as viruses and bacteria and move them out of the body.

Ginger is more Toxic to Breast Cancer Cells and Advanced Disease than Taxol

A pungent component within ginger known as 6-shogaol is superior to conventional chemotherapy in targeting the root cause of breast cancer malignancy: namely, the breast cancer stem cells.

Cancer stem cells are at the root of a wide range of cancers and are sometimes referred to as "mother cells" because they are responsible for producing all the different "daughter" cell types that makeup the tumor colony. While cancer stem cells only constitute between 0.2 and 1.0% of the cells within any given tumor, they seem to possess a virtually "immortal" ability to self-renew, are capable of continuous differentiation, are resistant to conventional chemotherapeutic agents, and are tumorigenic (i.e., are capable of "splitting off" to create new tumor colonies). Clearly, the cancer stem cells within a tumor must be destroyed if cancer treatment is to effect a lasting cure.

A new study titled, "6-Shogaol Inhibits Breast Cancer Cells and Stem Cell-Like Spheroids by Modulation of Notch Signaling Pathway and Induction of Autophagic Cell Death," identified powerful anti-cancer stem cell activity in 6-shogaol, a pungent constituent of ginger produced when the root is either dried or cooked. The study also found that the cancer-destroying effects occurred at concentrations that were non-toxic to non-cancerous cells – a crucial difference from conventional cancer treatments that do not provide this kind of selective cytotoxicity and therefore can do great harm to the patient.

Activator:

Protandim as a drug intended to prevent or treat diseases. Protandim supplements are Nrf1 and Nrf2. Nrf2 is found as a transcription factor as seen in EGCG (or green tea). Nrf2 nutrients are found in turmeric (curcumin), resveratrol in grape skin and berries (stilbenes), green tea and dark chocolate (catechins) and cruciferous veggies (isothiocyanates and sulforaphane). In the case of fast growing, chemo-resistant cancers, super high doses of these Nrf2 synergizer should be used along with other cancer therapy protocols to override the mutated Nrf2 pathways used by the cancer cells.[54] Protandim, a well-defined combination of widely studied medicinal plants, has been shown to induce superoxide dismutase (SOD) and catalase activities and reduce superoxide generation and lipid peroxidation in healthy human subjects.

Protandim prevents skin tumor formation via the induction of several primary antioxidant enzymes. As the induction of antioxidant enzymes is a much more potent approach than supplementation with conventional stoichiometric antioxidants.

Each of the five ingredients of Protandim shows anti-cancer effects and other activities:

1. **Bacosides**, a traditional Ayurvedic medicine, has been used in India for centuries as a memory enhancing, anti-inflammatory, analgesic, antipyretic, sedative, and antiepileptic agent.

2. **Silymarin** is known as a hepatoprotectant, but also shows anti-cancer and cytoprotective activities on organs, including the prostate, lungs, CNS, kidneys, pancreas and skin.

3. **W. somnifera** has shown anti-angiogenesis and anti-cancer activities.

4. **Green tea (EGCG)** shows promising results in cancer prevention and treatment in a large number of studies.

5. **Curcumin** is another rising star as a cancer prevention agent and decreases inflammation.

However, besides having a synergistic effect, the benefits of forming this combination include lowering the concentration of each ingredient to reduce any potential side effects.[55]

CANNABINOIDS

Pain

CBD Oil comes from cannabinoids and possesses anti-proliferative and pro-apoptotic effects. They are known to interfere with tumor neovascularization, cancer cell migration, adhesion, invasion, metastasizing, and decreases advanced disease.

CBD Oil decreases pain. It is cumulative, meaning it gives stronger pain relief as it is applied the longer it is used. CBD Oil does not depress the immune system, and may trigger cell-suicide in cancer cells. This action reduces tumor growth. CBD minimizes inflammation.

Remember that all prescription pain medication, except Tramadol, depresses the immune system. Google "every medication and the immune system" before you take them. CBD increases the immune system.

Take as directed.

Additional Cancer Treatments:

→ **Epigallocatechin gallate (ECGC) + Curcumin + Grape seed extract is a strong anticancer combination.**

→ **Laetrile or B17 or Amygdalin** (three different substances):

- **Amygdalin** is a natural substance that's found in raw nuts like almonds and the seeds and kernels of many fruits, particularly apricots. It's also present in lima beans, clover, sorghum and many other things.
- **Vitamin B-17** is the name given this substance by Dr. Ernst T. Krebs Jr., the man who first identified amygdalin. He called it a food component. Food components are natural, non-toxic, water-soluble and compatible with human metabolisms.
- **Laetrile** is the concentrated, purified form of amygdalin developed for use in the laboratory and in cancer treatment.

Laetrile is believed to fight cancer by targeting and killing cancer cells while building the immune system to fend off future outbreaks. Amygdalin is made up of glucose plus two potentially toxic substances – benzaldehyde and hydrogen cyanide.

Healthy cells contain the enzyme rhodanese which protects the cells by neutralizing the benzaldehyde and cyanide in amygdalin, converting them to useful nutrient compounds, including thiocyanate, which is known as a natural regulator of blood pressure and is also involved in the production of vitamin B-12.

Cancer cells do not have rhodanese. Instead, they have an enzyme called beta-glucosidase. Beta-glucosidase unlocks the benzaldehyde and cyanide from the glucose to create a targeted poison that kills the cancer cell.[56]

◈ **Paw paw** is 24x stronger than the leading graviola product.
According to Dr. Jerry McLaughlin of Purdue University, Asimina triloba, a type of paw paw, was significantly effective in battling cancer cells, as well as parasites, insects such as lice, and other invaders. Paw paw leaves eliminated lung, pancreatic and prostate cancer cells.

Paw paw contains natural chemicals called acetogenins, which are long-chained fatty acids that produce adenosine triphosphate (ATP) in cancer cells, and which diminish the growth of blood vessels that feed nutrients to the cells. It also slows the growth of multiple drug resistance (MDR) cells. Paw paw is the only cancer treatment—natural or otherwise—that has shown effectiveness against these types of cells.[57]

Graviola is not nearly as potent as Paw paw.
Take AIM **Barley Life**, an alkaline, in both pills and powder. Take about 6-20 pills each morning and drink 2 vegetable drinks, one in the morning and one in the afternoon.
Health Benefits of Barley Grass:

1. Has antioxidant power
2. Helps to relieve ulcerative colitis
3. Helps to boost the immune system
4. Acts as a natural detoxifier
5. Helps to Prevent Cancer
6. Protects against UV Radiation
7. Helps to reduce excess acidity
8. Helps to fight addiction
9. Helps to prevent signs of aging
10. Helps to repair DNA
11. Helps to boost red blood cell levels
12. Helps to relieve migraines

The consumption of barley grass is safe.

Fluoride

Fluoride has long been recognized as an enzyme inhibitor. Since the 1800s, fluoride has been a key component in rat poison and insecticides. When mixed into grain or other food, rats will readily consume the poison and die. This is mixed at 0.52ppm or 0.52 milligrams of fluoride in rat poison. This is less than is put in the water supply.

Water fluoridation is the process of adding fluoride to the water supply so the level reaches approximately 0.7 ppm, or 0.7 milligrams of fluoride per liter of water; this is the optimal level for preventing tooth decay. Fluoride is a poison! . . . it has been used as a pesticide for mice, rats and other small pests. A 10-pound infant could be killed by 1/100 of an ounce and a 100-pound adult could be killed by 1/10 of an ounce of fluoride.

People suffer from the intentional poisoning of human beings through accumulated fluoride toxicity from daily exposure.[58]

Fluoride is a proven neurotoxin; it causes birth defects, impairs the immune system, causes muscular weakness, gastrointestinal symptoms, and bone and joint symptoms; it suppresses thyroid function, and it causes permanent disfiguration of teeth.

Only distilled water gets rid of over 99% of fluoride in the cells. Drink half your body weight in ounces of water as well as the number of ounces for anything else you drink. For example, 12 ounces coffee requires 12 ounces water to offset dehydration. Only do this for four days, maximum.

I bathe with a Kangen water attachment that attaches to the shower to provide a fluoride free shower daily.

More Things to Avoid:

1) Microwaves produce harmful radiation and damage healthy nutrients
2) Dirty water—all water should be filtered.
3) Household Chemicals:
- Phthalates, found in many fragranced household products, such as air fresheners, dish soap—even toilet paper.
- Perchloroethylene or "PERC"
- Triclosan
- Quarternary Ammonium Compounds, or "QUATS"
- 2-Butoxyethanol
- Ammonia
- Chlorine
- Sodium Hydroxide

4) Non-organic makeup, shampoo, conditioner, hair spray, deodorant (no aluminum), soap, perfumes and anything else that touches your body. Anything that touches your body will be absorbed in 28 seconds.

Hormone Control

By controlling your blood glucose level and elevating your ketone levels you can begin to activate many beneficial hormones in your blood stream which promote healing. Low levels of insulin cause a release of beneficial hormones such as growth hormones and other powerful growth factors. While high levels of Cholesterol boost hormone levels, that may not be good for cancer growth as many cancers are hormone sensitive and actually grow in the presence of hormones. Melatonin balances hormones. Deceasing Melatonin levels cause increasing Breast cancer.

Myrrh is known to support healthy hormone balance, which is essential in cancer healing. Thyme also decreases hormones.

CHAPTER 8: ELECTRICITY AND ENERGY

"LORD, be gracious to us; we long for you. Be our strength every morning, our salvation in time of distress." - Isaiah 33:2

HOW SOUND, LIGHT AND ELECTRO-ENERGY CAN HEAL THE BODY

The human body is comprised of electro-magnetic transmissions and communication. The body sends out and receives electro-magnetic waves, this is energy. The electromagnetic energies that live in human tissue are very strong. When you send out energy to a living cell with the precise frequency that it needs, it will respond positively, and health can return in short order. **Whatever it is called hertz, voltage, frequency, chi, prana, chakras, it is all energy.**

The human body resonates at a frequency of 62-78 MHz and scientists believe that diseases start at 58 MHz. Many studies have shown that negative thoughts can reduce our frequency by 12 MHz, while positive thinking raises it by 10 MHz. But Hertz meters are only found in lab, but we can use a voltage meter to obtain measurements.

This means that there are many things that can affect our health in ways we can't imagine. According to the latest studies, essential oils can fight advanced disease because of antibacterial properties and their ability to change the energy at which we resonate.

One of the scientists involved in the study, Bruce Tainio, developed a special Calibrated Frequency Monitor that measures the frequency of essential oils and how they affect us. M. Suhail, an immunologist, says that cancer develops when the DNA in our cells' nucleus is corrupted.

Essential oils can correct this and repair the code, effectively improving our chances against dreadful disease.

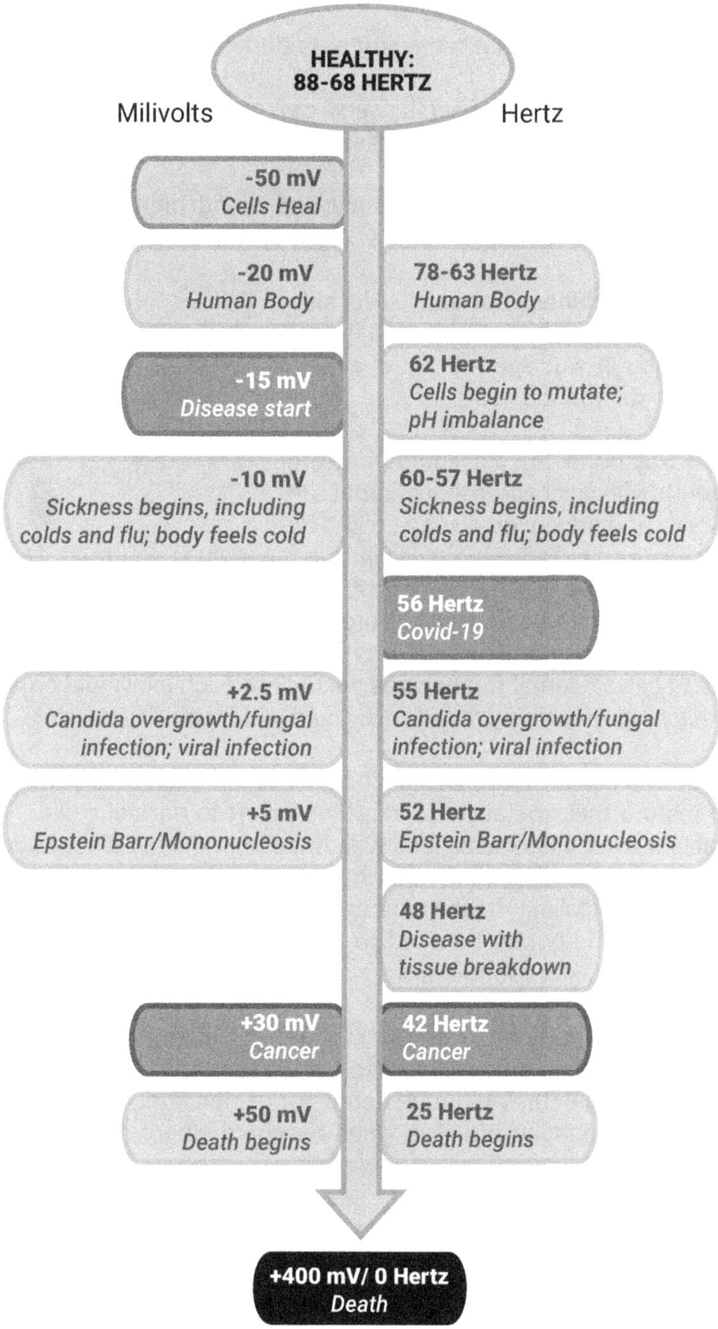
HEALTHY:
88-68 HERTZ
Milivolts
Hertz
-50 mV
Cells Heal
-20 mV
Human Body
78-63 Hertz
Human Body
-15 mV
Disease start
62 Hertz
Cells begin to mutate; pH imbalance
-10 mV
Sickness begins, including colds and flu; body feels cold
60-57 Hertz
Sickness begins, including colds and flu; body feels cold
56 Hertz
Covid-19
+2.5 mV
Candida overgrowth/fungal infection; viral infection
55 Hertz
Candida overgrowth/fungal infection; viral infection
+5 mV
Epstein Barr/Mononucleosis
52 Hertz
Epstein Barr/Mononucleosis
48 Hertz
Disease with tissue breakdown
+30 mV
Cancer
42 Hertz
Cancer
+50 mV
Death begins
25 Hertz
Death begins
+400 mV/ 0 Hertz
Death

In his book, *The Body Electric*, R. O. Becker said that our bodies' electronic frequency or energy determines our health.

Even Nikola Tesla said that removing outside frequencies or energy can make us more resistant to ailments, while Dr. Otto Warburg discovered over a century ago that our cells have a specific electrical voltage that can drop due to a various factors and trigger diseases such as cancer.[59]

I recommend replacing low frequency and using higher frequency or energy machines.

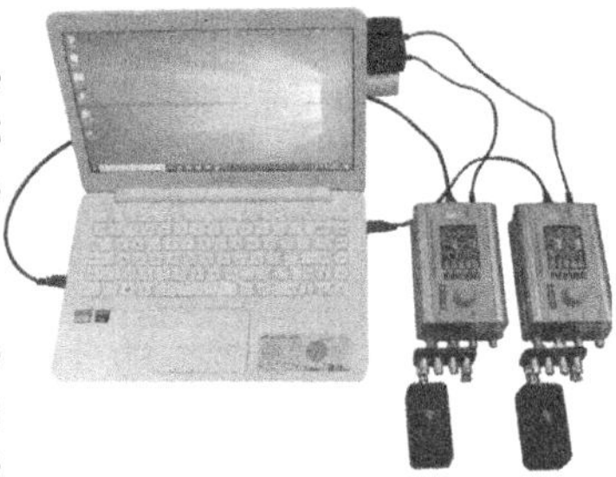

a. **Rife machines**—portable. No side effects are likely as most machines in the US have low enough wattage that there are no issues. It costs about $1,000.

Dr. Royal Raymond Rife invented the Rife Machine. Dr. Rife discovered that microbes in cancer cells and advanced disease could be totally devitalized by radio energies which left patients unharmed. His work culminated with The Smithsonian Institution publishing the following quote in their 1944 annual report: "Disease organisms such those of tuberculosis, cancer, sarcoma, typhoid, and others may be observed to succumb when exposed to certain lethal frequencies peculiar to each individual organism, and directed upon them by rays conveying a wide range of waves."

It is possible to kill the microbes inside of the cells, which allows the cancer cells to restore their metabolism and thus revert to normal cells. This is the ideal way to attack disease because there are no dead disease cells to create a Herxheimer reaction[60] that must be eliminated by detoxification of the body. This killing off the cancer cells without die off prevents poor reactions. Electricity can be used to kill cancer quickly as building the immune system takes a longer time.[61]

Microorganisms (pathogens and microbes), including viruses, bacteria, and fungi each have a specific vibration or signature to which they can be exposed, resulting in their ultimate death or deactivation. The best way to describe this resonating effect is when an opera singer shatters a glass with the right pitch, carried by audio waves.

While in every disease situation, frequency generators can be an effective component of the treatment, there are special situations which are critical for reenergizing the body.

1) The patient cannot digest foods effectively (usually due to stomach or

colon surgery), thus nutritional protocols may not be effective enough.

2) The patient cannot extract nutrients from foods, which happens when the lining of the stomach is damaged by chemotherapy or other medications.

3) The patient has a very fast-growing disease which means they need every advantage possible to stop its spread.

4) Disease has spread throughout the body, in which case they need a strong multi-pronged attack.

5) There is cancer in their bones or bone marrow and nutritional protocols may not be able to reach the cancer cells.

6) The patient would be put at risk if inflammation and swelling were experienced due to the treatment. Frequency or electrical generators, which have a carrier energy, work better to kill microbes inside of cells (which allows the cells to revert to normal cells), there is no inflammation caused by dying cells.

7) Their type of disease involves massive infections (though the type of microbe must be identified) to run the correct frequency or energy.

b. **Photon Genius** – It costs about $27,00.00. It is not portable. No side effects are likely as most machines in the US have low enough wattage that there are no issues.

The Photon Genius is essentially an Energy-Medicine Instrument that provides the following energies and therapies for use by the human body:

- Electrical Energy
- Electro-magnetic Energy
- Bio-Photonic Energy
- Frequency Harmonics
- Energy Infrared Transmission
- Proprietary Noble Gas Technology
- Heat Therapy
- Sauna Therapy
- Anti-oxidative Therapy Light Therapy
- Sound Therapy
- Nitric Oxide Therapy
- Detoxification

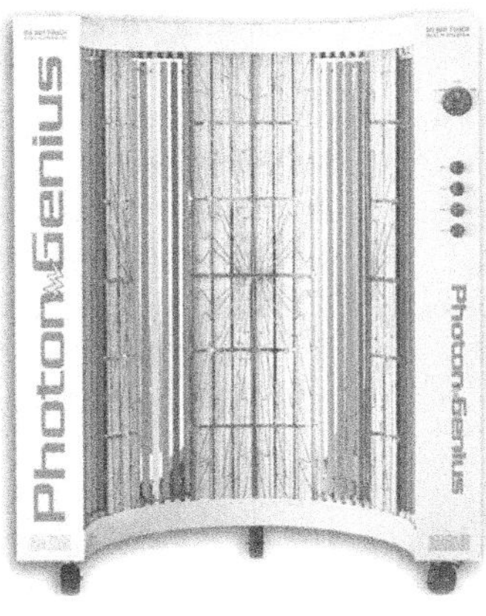

c. **Photon Genie** – It costs about $4,000.00 – much less than above, but on a much smaller scale. It is portable. No side effects are likely as most machines in the US are low enough wattage that there are no issues.

The Photon Genie does the following:

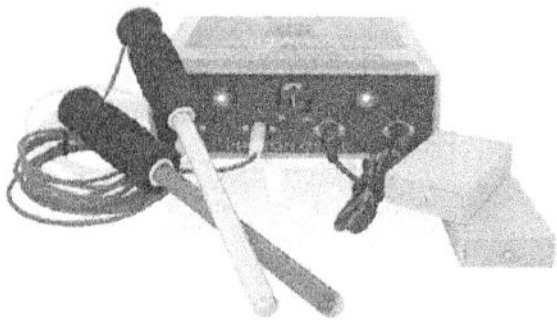

1. Stimulating and strengthening the immune system.
2. Reducing and eliminating pain.
3. Ozonating and Oxygenating the body.
4. Moving and balancing fluid systems of the body through all the channels (blood vessels, lymph, capillaries) for the transport of nutrition and vital energy and the proper management of toxins by the body.
5. Devitalizing pathogens (viruses, bacteria, fungus, parasites, mold, yeast), clearing infections, slowing and reversing disease processes.
6. Eliminating blockages by repolarizing cells and molecules; dissolving lumps, clots, mineral deposits, etc.
7. Revitalizing the body by moving all the fluids (lymph, blood, etc.).
8. Reestablishing the cells' normal vibrational balance and energizing the cellular state.
9. Neutralizing negative "thought-forms" and stagnant energy patterns that compound over long periods of time being sick and fatigued.
10. Increasing energy levels and providing a sense of well-being, relaxation, clarity and relief.
11. Recharging life-force energy at the cellular level and facilitating higher and clearer states of awareness.
12. Athletically increasing and maintaining consistent peak performance without interruption from muscle stress, strain and injuries.
13. Complete Veterinary application: dramatic, rapid, reliable, lifesaving results with pets; a must for all animal lovers.
14. Cosmetic uses for more youthful skin toning and regeneration, without painful and costly surgery.
15. Accelerating the removal of fat and cellulite, when used in conjunction with long-term exercise and proper diet.
16. Alleviate symptoms of PMS and menopause, including pain, irritability, bloating, depression, migraines, and hot flashes through hormone balancing.
17. Encouraging weight loss by neutralizing and balancing appetite cravings and increasing cellular energy levels.
18. Universal tool for complete photobiotic nutrition at the cell level, ideally used in conjunction with a more complete natural-health program.[62]

d. **Orgone Accumulator**[63] - $30.00 - It is portable. No side effects are likely as blankets have low enough wattage that there are no issues.

Wilheim Reich's developed the Orgone Accumulator. Using his research, the accumulator device charges the person situated inside with what he called, "orgone energy". He and his co-workers began an experimental program of treatment free-of-charge to the patients who were seriously diseased people.

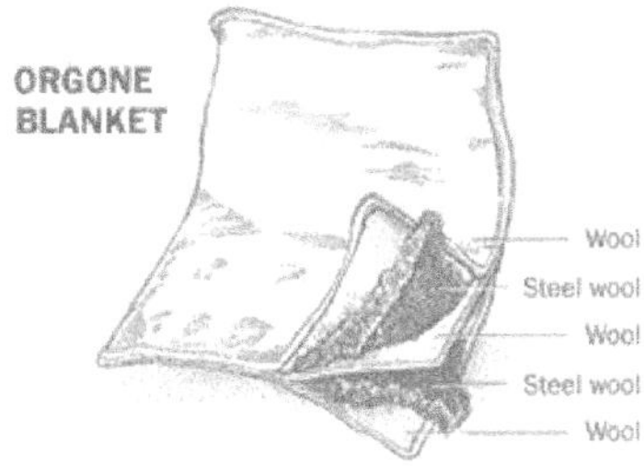

Dramatic changes in general condition, and positive influences were objectively documented in many patients, for such different disease processes as anemia, diabetes mellitus, various kinds of carcinoma and the acceleration of wound-healing processes. Experiments with humans as well as laboratory mice proved the orgone accumulator's value for the support of organic mechanisms of regulation and healing.

I made my own Orgone Accumulator blanket using 2 yards of 100% wool and steel wool purchased at Lowe's. Lay the wool on the floor and line one half of the wool with the steel wool, I used candles to mark about 4-inch rows of the steel wool. Fold the other side of the wool over the steel wool and then in half. Sew the lines where the candles were. Sew the edges of the wool. Make a Pillow case of 100% cotton to cover the wool blanket as it will be too scratchy without one.

e. **Biocharger**—It is not Portable.
No side effects are likely as most machines in the US are low enough that there are no issues. It costs about $15,000.

The transmitted energy stimulates and invigorates the entire body to optimize and improve potential health, wellness, and athletic performance. The BioCharger™ NG is completely non-invasive, and has been proven to restore strength, stamina, coordination and mental clarity. BioCharger™ NG helps to accelerate muscle recovery and reduce stiffness in joints. It also contributes to improved mobility and flexibility.[64]

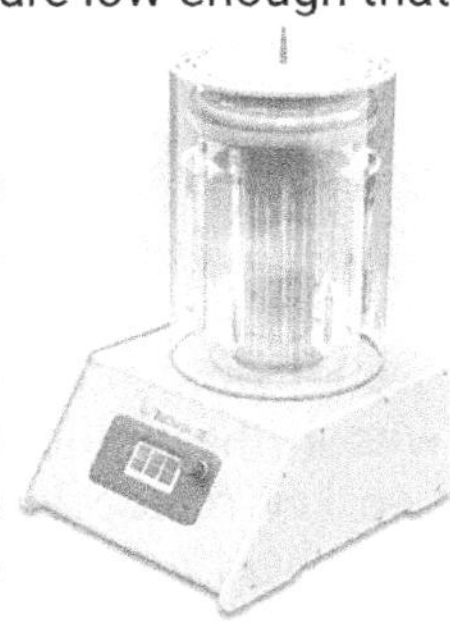

f. **Bob Beck Protocol**[65] —Portable. Four Machines in total. No side effects are likely as most machines in the US have low enough wattage that there are no issues. It costs about $1,000.

SilverPulser DC Electric[66]

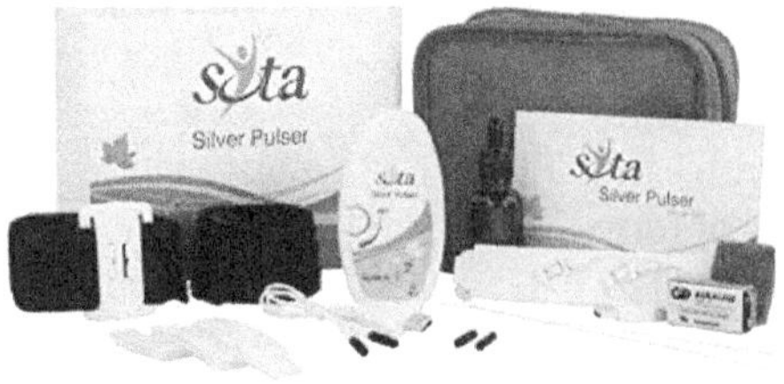

MicroPulser AC Electric[67]

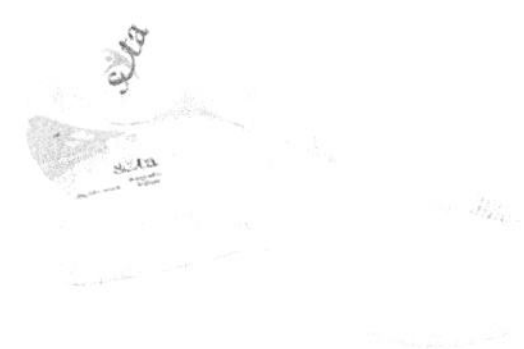

Colloidal Silver

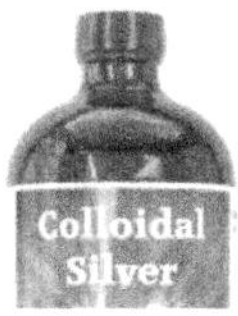

Ozonator[68]

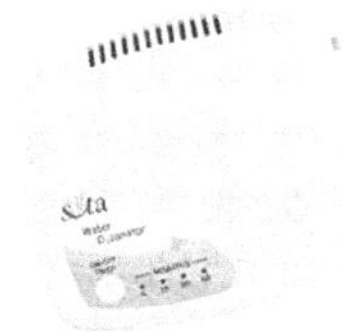

The Bob Beck (electromedicine) Protocol, strengthens the immune system, and is a potent alternative disease treatment. One way it works is by lowering the level of pathogens in the body which in turn helps the immune system to do its job.

Until now, no one knew the full potential of the immune system because every scientific study ever conducted on the immune system was on humans who had two pounds of disease-causing microbes (pathogens) in their bloodstream. Their immune systems were choked by these pathogens so no one had a clue how potent the immune system could be.

The late Dr. Bob Beck, a physicist with a doctoral degree in science, figured out a way to rid the body of pathogens. His discovery was actually based on the discovery of two medical doctors who were researching AIDS at the Albert Einstein College of Medicine.

What Dr. Beck learned is that, as you rid your body of pathogens, the immune system immediately begins to be supercharged. The specific section of the immune system that Dr. Beck suspected was supercharged was in the production of neuropeptides. The immune system creates two key molecules called interleukin and interferon. These molecules are called neuropeptides or nerve proteins. There are more than 2,000 neuropeptides in the body, but for the most part, their cancer-fighting effects are unknown. It may be that interleukin and interferon are not the most potent cancer-fighting neuropeptides. Neuropeptides are absolutely deadly to cancer and disease cells!

The Bob Beck Protocol, by getting rid of pathogens, allows these neuropeptides to be created in much higher volumes and the immune system is supercharged far beyond the imagination of scientists. This protocol should be taken very seriously.

g. **Solaragem**[69]—Portable. No side effects likely as this is a crystal light machine, not frequency, there are no reported issues. Costs about $750 with attachment crystals.

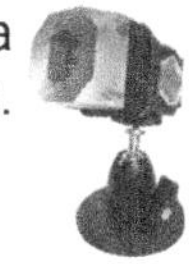

The Solaragem, known as Crystal Light Therapy, provides the wellness and balance on an emotional, mental, physical and spiritual level. It is defined as a therapeutic physical modality using photons to promote pain relief, tissue repair and increased circulation.

For rogue cancer cells to become dominant and spread through the body, the immune system needs to be in a state of high suppression, which can be a result of a range of negative factors on the mental, emotional, spiritual, and physical level. The Solaragem is a unique, vigorous hammer-and- sweep action which delivers an energy frequency to the body that eliminates these trace driver conditions from the body. It has been designed to support clients undergoing traditional and integrative cancer care and may be considered as a preventative tool to eradicate build-up of these trace driver conditions.

h. **Qest 4**[70]—The Qest4 system is a diagnostic tool loaded with over 40,000 homeopathic, nutritional, herbal, and pharmaceutical items for rapid energetic evaluation of their potential effectiveness. An integrated hardware test plate also enables energetically tested individual products that your client is currently using. It is portable. No side effects are likely this is a 2.6 V machine. There are no reported issues.

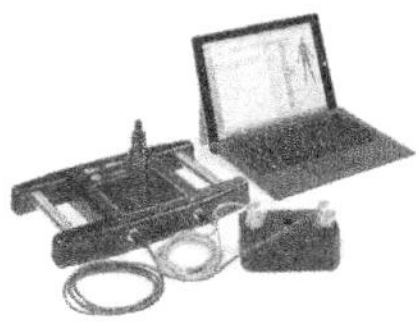

i. **Halo**—a unique, energetic device that harnesses the power of both plants and light to provide holistic comfort to the body. It is portable. It costs about $5,000.

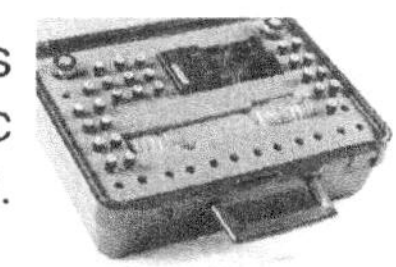

j. **Bemer**[71]—It is portable. It costs about $5,000.

The Bemer is great for situations in which a vascular blockage is known to exist.

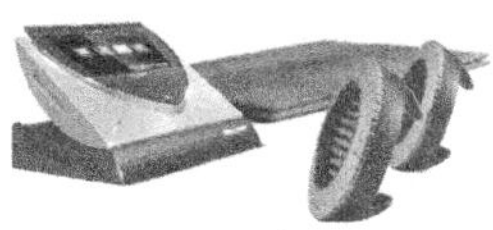

Bemer Physical Vascular Therapy improves microcirculation and promotes the blood flow in the smallest blood vessels.

This improves the performance of the body's cells, which in turn activates the body's own self-healing powers.

k. **Biomat and Biomat mini**[72]—Helps to release stress and detoxify the body. Simply lying on the BioMat promotes a feeling of well-being for a healthier mind and body. It costs about $2,000.

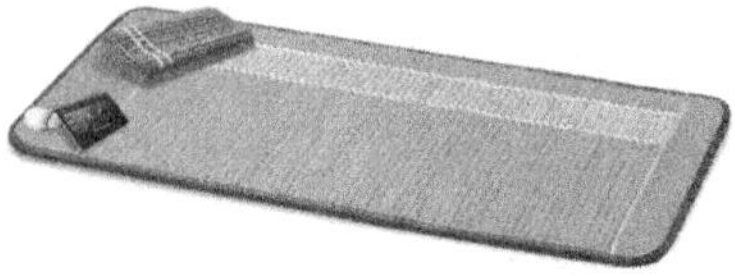

Benefits of the BioMat:

- Reduces stress and fatigue
- Relieves anxiety and promotes relaxation
- Improves sleep patterns
- Reduces inflammation
- Eases joint pain and stiffness
- Provides warm, soothing pain relief
- Eliminates toxins in the body
- Increases blood circulation
- Alleviates migraines and tension headaches
- Reduces allergy symptoms
- Improves immune system function
- Improves cardiovascular health
- Burns calories and controls weight
- Improves muscle tone and skin quality

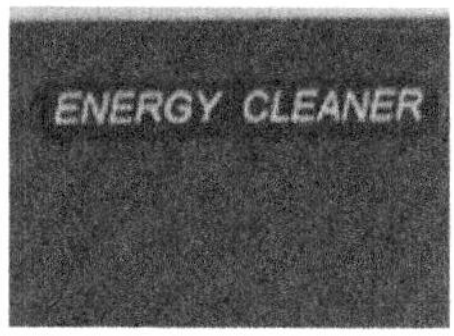

l. **Energy Cleaner** - hooks to an electric mattress pad (or can charge bath water), to be slept on each night. The EC causes a normal 24-hour detox to be completed every 6 minutes, or when the blood completely circulates through the liver.

Information Energy Chips AkuRy[73]

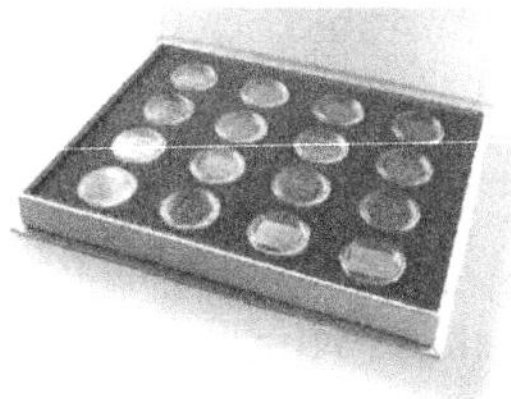

I use the Information Chips every day to maintain my health. You can get a quality product from Germany endorsed by Dr. Charles Krebs. He utilizes several of these chips in his practice, which are able to instantly decompensate numerous levels of stress. Many therapists, physicians and alternative practitioners use a complete set of chips for rapid assessment and to assist in treatment. The chips have a supportive effect.

The creator of the chip states: The chips must be activated "(10-15 seconds in your hand or place it on a specific place on the body intuitively). The operation of the chips is similar to a CD. If you simply look at a CD, you cannot see anything; however, there is information stored on it. Only once installed into a player does this information become audible or visible. In our case, the player is our body. The chips operate on the principle of resonance – our body only processes the frequencies or energies it needs. Overcharging will not occur.

Hydrogen Water

H2 (hydrogen water) is water with dissolved hydrogen and is said to reduce oxidative stress. Hydrogen machines cost more than $1,000, or bottles of water cost about $3, while hydrogen tablets can be dissolved in water to increase hydrogen content.

Some of these companies claim that adding more hydrogen to water increases your energy, improves recovery after exercise and reduces inflammation.

Alkaline water restores the body to wellness where it operates best, while hydrogen water has antioxidant effects. Use Alkaline water to heal.

Alkaline water	VS Hydrogen water
Increases Hydration	Decreases Free Radicals/Antioxidant Rich
Increases Performance and Decreases Fatigue	Decreases Blood Pressure
Increases Minerals	Increases Circulation
Increases Gut Health	Detoxes
Disinfects/Kills Microbes	Protects from Sunlight
Fights Chemical Buildup	Promotes Good Health
Decreases Risk of Diabetes	Increases Energy
Protects Body	Increases Collagen Production

Ozonator

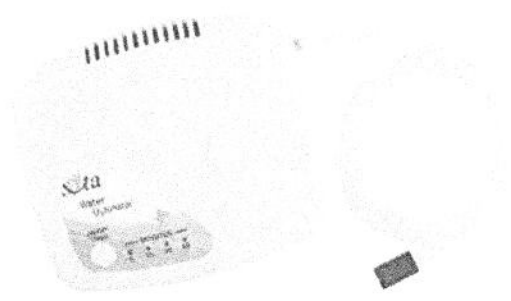

Ozonation Process

The transformation of oxygen into ozone occurs with the use of an electric discharge field. Ozone may also be made through electrolytic and chemical reactions. The raw water is then passed through a venturi throat which creates a vacuum and pulls the ozone gas into the water. It then bubbles up through the water being treated.

Ozone-treated water provides an oxygen-rich extracellular environment which decreases disease growth, as disease grows slowly in the presence of oxygen.

CHAPTER 9:
EXERCISE

"Praise the LORD, my soul, and forget not all his benefits, who forgives all your sins and heals all your diseases, who redeems your life from the pit and crowns you with love and compassion." - Psalms 103:2-4

Initially, exercise should not be so strenuous as to produce lactic acid which is the chemical that makes you sore.

To reduce lactic acid production – WALK. Lactic Acid is one way that cancer and advanced disease grows. According to Melanie Aichele, exercise releases the "hope" hormone. Regular exercise helps you rebuild your body by improving strength, endurance (fatigue) and confidence.

Try to increase a daily schedule of walking to 2-3 miles per day. Initially, walking may have to be limited to short periods of time until you are able to build up to 2-3 miles per day.

Walk, only, for the first three months. Additionally, add any low impact sports such as swimming. Then gradually add more strenuous exercise as your body becomes acclimated. This is a very individual determination.

CHAPTER 10: BEING HEALTHY AGAIN

"Dear friend, I pray that you may enjoy good health and that all may go well with you, even as your soul is getting along well." - 3 John 1:2

Being healthy again involves body, mind, and spirit. As your body heals, you must concentrate on healing the mind. "Survivor's guilt" must also be dealt with. Energy healing and Kinesiology will help release toxic misconceptions that you may have.

Spiritual issues are best dealt with through reading your Bible and praying. A minister to talk to will help. Go to church (or other place of worship) as being part of a larger religious group will help ground your spiritual issues and give you a support group.

Use humor to laugh and heal. Laughter puts your body in an ab alkaline state of being.

Wellness = nutrition + supplements + detoxing + exercise.

BIBLIOGRAPHY

a. No author name, written by Trinity School of Natural Health, Analyzing pH, no City noted, no printer noted, 2015, book.
b. No author name, written by Trinity School of Natural Health, Dried Blood Cell Analysis, no City noted, printed by Whitman Publications, 2017, book.
c. Wikipedia.
d. Ralph W. Moss, PhD, Cancer Coach, Article.
e. Robert Wright, Killing Cancer Not People, What I Would Do If I Had Cancer, 2nd Edition, American Anti-Cancer Institute, 2011, book.
f. Dr. Barry Richardson, Dean of the College of Business at Centenary College, in Shreveport Louisiana, where Diana received her Master of Business degree.
g. David Servan-Schreiber, Anticancer, Penguin Books, 2008, Book, page 21 footnote, Stephen Jay Gould, "The Median is Not the Message", Article.

ENDNOTES

[1]*The Chemistry of Man, page 261. (page 9)*

[2]*Analyzing pH, page 32. (page 9)*

[3] *Dried Blood Cell Analysis, page 10. (page 9)*

[4] *Ralph W. Moss, Article. (page 9)*

[5] *Analyzing pH, pages 5, 48. (page 10)*

[6] *The Chemistry of Man (page 10)*

[7]*Killing Cancer, Not People, page 25. (page 18)*

[8]*The Chemistry of Man, page 297. (page 20)*

[9]*Analyzing pH, page 57. (page 20)*

[10] *Dried Blood Cell Analysis, page 19-20. (page 20)*

[11]*Analyzing pH, page 48. (page 25)*

[12]*David Servan-Schreiber, Anticancer, Penguin Books, 2008, Book, footnote page 21, Stephen Jay Gould, "The Median is Not the Message", Article. (page 30)*

[13]*Analyzing pH, page 12. (page 31)*

[14] *American Cancer Society (page 41)*

[15] *Holtord Medical Group. What is a Herxheimer Reaction and What Can I Do About It? in El Segundo CA & Marietta GA. (2020). https://www.holtorfmed.com/what-is-a-herxheimer-reaction-and-what-can-i-do-about-it/ (page 42)*

[16]*Dr. Donna Schwontkowski. 40 Signs You Need A Colon Cleanse & 4 Steps*

To Clean It Fast. (2021). https://www.nutracraft.com/blogs/colon/40-signs-you-need-a-colon-cleanse-4-steps-to-clean-it-fast (page 47)

[17] *Catherin Rudolph. 10 Signs of a Clogged Lymphatic System and 20 Ways To Cleanse It - Foods That Heal You. (2016). https://foodsthathealyou.com/20-ways-to-drain-your-lymph/ (page 47)*

[18] *Dr. Richard Gerhauser, MD, The Secrets of Underground Medicine, page 136-137. (page 50)*

[19] *A Quick-Start 24-Hour Liver Cleanse by Dr Axe. (2019). https://chocolatree.com/blogs/news/a-quick-start-24-hour-liver-cleanse-by-dr-axe (page 51)*

[20] *Judy Seeger, N. (2017). How to effectively detox after cancer treatments - Cancer Tutor. https://www.cancertutor.com/detoxing-after-cancer-treatments/ (page 56)*

[21] *Korin Miller & Bindiya Gandhi 10 Signs You May Have A Parasite. (2013). https://www.mindbodygreen.com/articles/intestinal-parisites-signs-symptoms-and-how-to-get-rid-of-them (page 57)*

[22] *Tiffany Rowen, created the Petrochemical Protocol (page 60)*

[23] *Note: Each person must buy their own array which is the detoxing personal part of the footbath. (page 60)*

[24] *Allopathic Treatment is traditional Chemical Medicine of doctors and nurses, it is chemotherapy, radiation and surgery with many side effects. (page 61)*

[25] *Late Effects of Cancer Treatment. (2016) https://www.livestrong.org/we-can-help/healthy-living-after-treatment/late-effects-of-cancer-treatment (page 61)*

[26] *A diet of 80% fresh vegetables and juice, whole grains, seeds, nutsnuts, and a little fruit s help put the body into an alkaline state. 20% can be from cooked food, including beans. Fresh vegetable juices provide live enzymes that are easily absorbed and get down to cellular levels within 15 minutes to nourish and enhance growth of healthy cells. (page 63)*

[27] *Dilute essential oils in a carrier oil such as olive oil. Use three to five drops of essential oil for each ounce of carrier oil. Herbal remedies could provide other health benefits alongside pain-relieving effects, such as having antioxidant effects to help keep the body healthy. (page 64)*

[28] Chemotherapy most likely to cause mouth sores are:, Capecitabine (Xeloda), Cisplatin, Cytarabine (Depocyt), Doxorubicin (Doxil), Etoposide (Etopophos), Fluorouracil, Methotrexate (Trexall). Everolimus (Afinitor) is a targeted therapy drug that stimulates the immune system to fight cancer. I, it can produce mouth sores as a side effect. Aa mouth rinse, using the drug dexamethasone, can help prevent mouth sores in people receiving the targeted drug everolimus, according to the Mayo Clinic. (page 68)

[29] Reference Guide for Essential Oils by Connie and Alan Higley, 2014 Edition, Abundant Health. (page 73)

[30] Your post-cancer treatment sex Rx, By Diane Mapes/ Fred Hutch News Service. Diane Mapes is a staff writer at Fred Hutchinson Cancer Research Center. She has written extensively about health issues for NBC News, TODAY, CNN, MSN, Seattle Magazine and other publications. A breast cancer survivor, she blogs at doublewhammied.com and tweets@double_whammied. Email her at dmapes@fredhutch.org. (page 76)

[31]Dana-Farber Cancer Institute. Your Body after Treatment. https://www.dana-farber.org/for-patients-and-families/for-survivors/caring-for-yourself-after-cancer/your-body-after-treatment/ (page 79)

[32] A, S., V, A., & C, A. (2005). Cancer stem cells. Neoplasma, 52(6). https://www.ncbi.nlm.nih.gov/pubmed/16284686 (page 80)

[33] Rogel Cancer Center. Cancer Stem Cell Research. (2013). https://www.rogelcancercenter.org/research/stem-cells (page 80)

[34] Killing Cancer Not People page 146 (page 84)

[35] I did not have time to verify everything when I had Stage 4 Ovarian Cancer, so I would have to trust that certain individuals were accurate. I felt that Robert Wright's review of water was accurate. (page 85)

[36] 2009 study published in the journal Cancer Research (page 86)

[37] According to Dr. Ed Group (page 87)

[38] Similar to Bulletproof Coffee (page 92)

[39] https://genechanger.com/black-cumin-seed-oil-targets-cancer/ (page 92)

[40]Grape Seed Effective for Combating Cancer? What The Research Says. (2021).https://primalherb.com/grape-seed-is-surprisingly-effective-for-

beating-cancer/ (page 100)

[41] *B vitamins - Wikipedia. (2021). https://en.wikipedia.org/wiki/B_vitamins (page 101)*

[42]*Rady, I., Mohamed, H., Rady, M., Siddiqui, I., & Mukhtar, H. (2018). Cancer preventive and therapeutic effects of EGCG, the major polyphenol in green tea. Egyptian Journal Of Basic And Applied Sciences, 5(1), 1-23. doi: 10.1016/j.ejbas.2017.12.001*
https://www.sciencedirect.com/science/article/pii/S2314808X1730533X (page 104)

[43]*William Faloon. CoQ10 and Cancer Treatment. https://www.lifeextension.com/Magazine/2009/9/CoQ10-And-Cancer-Treatment/Page-01 (page 104)*

[44]*Kaplan, B. (2018). Anticancer Properties of Omega-3 Fatty Acids: Plant-Based vs Marine-Based - Oncology Nurse Advisor.*
https://www.oncologynurseadvisor.com/home/cancer-types/breast-cancer/anticancer-properties-of-omega-3-fatty-acids-plant-based-vs-marine-based/
(page 104)

[45] *Melissa Conrad Stopple. Medical Definition of Selenium (2021) https://www.medicinenet.com/script/main/art.asp?articlekey=5445 (page 105)*

[46] *Dr. Amanda Martin & Kirk Stokel. What Forms of Selenium Protect Against Cancer? (2020). https://www.lifeextension.com/magazine/2012/ss/selenium-protect-against-cancer/page-01 (page 105)*

[47] *Prasad, A., Beck, F., Snell, D., & Kucuk, O. (2009). Zinc in Cancer Prevention. Nutrition And Cancer, 61(6), 879-887. doi: 10.1080/01635580903285122*
https://www.ncbi.nlm.nih.gov/pubmed/20155630
(page 106)

[48] *Castiglioni, S., & Maier, J. (2011). Magnesium and cancer: a dangerous liason. Magnesium Research, 24(3), 92-100. doi: 10.1684/mrh.2011.0285*
https://www.ncbi.nlm.nih.gov/pubmed/21933757
(page 106)

[49]*Julia Greewald. Magnesium Deficiency and Cancer. (page 106)*

[50] *Elahe Motevaseli, S. (2017). The Role of Probiotics in Cancer Treatment: Emphasis on their In Vivo and In Vitro Anti-metastatic Effects. International Journal Of Molecular And Cellular Medicine, 6(2), 66.*
https://www.ncbi.nlm.nih.gov/pmc/articles/PMC5581548/ (page 107)

[51] Hao, F., Kumar, S., Yadav, N., & Chandra, D. (2014). Neem components as potential agents for cancer prevention and treatment. Biochimica Et Biophysica Acta (BBA) - Reviews On Cancer, 1846(1), 247-257. doi: 10.1016/j.bbcan.2014.07.002
https://www.ncbi.nlm.nih.gov/pmc/articles/PMC4734358/
(page 108)

[52]Brian Chomniak. Chlorella: A Cancer Killer Superfood. (2015).
https://breastcancerconqueror.com/chlorella-a-cancer-killer-superfood/
(page 109)

[53] Franco-Molina, M., Mendoza-Gamboa, E., Sierra-Rivera, C., Gómez-Flores, R., Zapata-Benavides, P., & Castillo-Tello, P. et al. (2010). Antitumor activity of colloidal silver on MCF-7 human breast cancer cells. Journal Of Experimental & Clinical Cancer Research, 29(1). doi: 10.1186/1756-9966-29-148
https://www.ncbi.nlm.nih.gov/pmc/articles/PMC2996348/ (page 110)

[54] Protandim® Nrf2 Synergizer® | LifeVantage United States (en)*
"Protandim® Nrf2 Synergizer® | Lifevantage United States (En)". United States (En), 2021, https://drdianawright.lifevantage.com/us-en/shop/protandim-nrf2. Accessed 7 Dec 2021. (page 111)*

[55]Liu, J., Gu, X., Robbins, D., Li, G., Shi, R., McCord, J., & Zhao, Y. (2009). Protandim, a Fundamentally New Antioxidant Approach in Chemoprevention Using Mouse Two-Stage Skin Carcinogenesis as a Model. Plos ONE, 4(4), e5284. doi: 10.1371/journal.pone.0005284
https://journals.plos.org/plosone/article?id=10.1371/journal.pone.0005284
(page 111)

[56] Vitamin B-17 vs. Laetrile - Everything You Need to Know. (2013). https://www.cancertutor.com/laetrile/ (page 112)

[57] Daily, T. (2013). Paw Paw and Graviola: Two Potent Anti-Cancer Trees.
https://www.thealternativedaily.com/paw-paw-the-miracle-anti-cancer-tree/
(page 113)

[58] Ty Bollinger. Events, T., Cancer Causes, T., Causes, C., Prevention, C., Treatments, C., & Drink, F. et al. (2021). Fluoride—Drinking Ourselves to Death?.
https://thetruthaboutcancer.com/fluoride-drinking-ourselves-to-death/
(page 114)

[59] Edzard Ernst. Here's What Oncologists Won't Tell You About Essential Oils. (2018). https://edzardernst.com/2018/05/heres-what-oncologists-wont-tell-you-about-essential-oils/ (page 118)

[60] *Herxheimer reaction is an increase in the symptoms of a spirochetal disease (as syphilis, Lyme disease, or relapsing fever) occurring in some persons treated with spirocheticidal drugs. https://www.merriam-webster.com/medical/Jarisch-Herxheimer%20reaction. (page 118)*

[61] *This technology and the scientific principles and physics involved are chronicled in the 2 videos: The Royal Rife Story and Royal Rife: In His Own Words (page 118)*

[62] *Ed Skilling Institute for Technology. A Fresh Perspective on Health Photon Genie Electromedicine. http://centerforinquiry.org/wp-content/uploads/sites/33/quackwatch/photon_genie.pdf (page 120)*

[63] *The Daily Omnivore. Orgone. (2012). https://thedailyomnivore.net/2012/10/24/orgone/ (page 121)*

[64] *https://biocharger.com/hybrid-serp/?gclid=EAIaIQobChMIrLrSv5j43wIVC77ACh3etw-yEAAYASAAEgLkavD_BwE (page 121)*

[65] *Research, F. The Official Bob Beck Site — The Beck Protocol. (2021). https://www.bobbeck.com/ (page 121)*

[66] *Sota. The Silver Pulser. (2021). https://www.sota.com/default.aspx?page=Silver-Pulser (page 122)*

[67] *Sota. The Magnetic Pulser. (2021). https://www.sota.com/default.aspx?page=Magnetic-Pulser (page 122)*

[68] *Sota. The Water O3zonator. (2021). https://www.sota.com/default.aspx?page=Water-Ozonator (page 122)*

[69] *SolaraGem Crystal Fusion Light*
"Solaragem Crystal Fusion Light". Solaragem.Com, 2021, https://solaragem.com/. Accessed 7 Dec 2021. (page 123)

[70] *Understanding Qest4 Testing - Qest4 Bioenergetic Health System. (2021). https://www.qest4.co.uk/understanding-qest4-testing/ (page 123)*

[71] *Product | Improve Functional Microcirculation | BEMER Life. (2021). https://life.bemergroup.com/product/#features (page 123)*

[72] *Biomat Direct. Richway - Biomat Professional 7000MX 74"x28." (2021) https://biomatdirect.com/products/richway-biomat-professional-7000mx-74x28 (page 124)*

[73] *Akury GmbH. Akury - Produktinformationen - akury. (2021). https://www.akuryprodukte.de/produktinformationen/ (page 124)*

Diana's Documentary

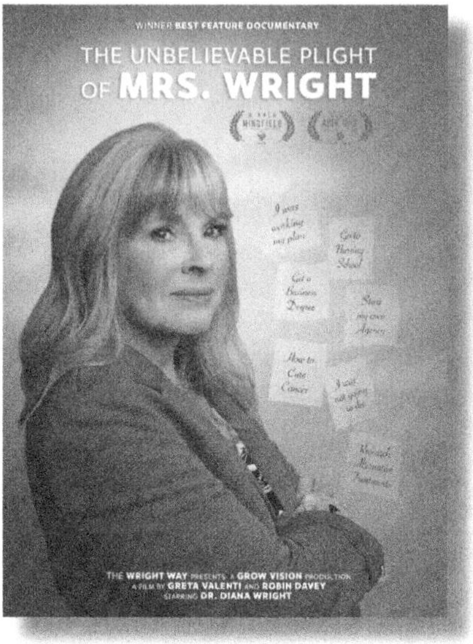

THE UNBELIEVABLE PLIGHT OF MRS. WRIGHT

Watch the incredible true story of American nurse and entrepreneur, Diana Wright. Overcoming poverty and abuse, Wright built a multi-million dollar business devoted to improving the quality of life for nurses, only to be given a terminal cancer death sentence by the very industry she dedicated her life to. Failed by the American medical system with only eight months to live, Diana takes her health into her own hands, spending her forecasted time in search of the cure for cancer.

Available on

amazon

Visit the Official Movie Site at

WWW.PLIGHTOFMRSWRIGHT.COM

DIRECTED BY GROW VISION STUDIOS

GROW VISION

Made in the USA
Las Vegas, NV
16 March 2026

43738905R00075